WHAT PEOPLE ARE SAYING ABOUT
YOU'RE PREGNANT, NOW WHAT?

•••

"Moms will truly relate to this book in various ways. I keep nodding my head in sheer agreement chapter after chapter, all while remembering how it was like during my pregnancies and the first year with my children. Katina delivers this book with a great sense of humour and an honest approach to being a mom."
Lyne Proulx (Founder, Ottawa Mommy Club)

•••

"As a parent, I know the helpless feeling as well as the feeling of losing your mind ... It is so wonderful that you are sharing your story so that moms can reach out for help without feeling like they are being judged."
J. Thompson (Ottawa)

•••

"Good tips. I could have used some of these with my oldest. I spent hours and hours holding him and rocking him."
Christine N. (Ottawa)

•••

"There are portions of the material that made me laugh out loud as I read as I recalled similar absurdities we endured."
Josephine Beddia (Montreal)

YOU'RE PREGNANT, NOW WHAT?

The good, the bad, and the ugly of pregnancy and baby's first year

•••

KATINA MICHELIS, M.Sc.

Published by Working Girl Press
4472 Shoreline Drive
Ottawa, Ontario K1V 1S7
(613) 298-2169

Library and Archives Canada Cataloguing in Publication

Michelis, Katina, 1973-, author
    You're pregnant, now what? : the good, the bad, and the ugly of pregnancy and baby's first year / Katina Michelis.

Issued in print and electronic formats.
ISBN 978-1-926958-26-2 (pbk.).-- ISBN 978-1-926958-27-9 (pdf)

    1. Pregnancy--Popular works. 2. Childbirth--Popular works. 3. Infants--Care--Popular works. I. Title.

RG525.M52 2013   618.2   C2013-902585-5
                              C2013-902586-3

Cover design by Sundus Asif
Author photograph by Jerry Ferentinos

For Ted, Eva, and Gia.
My family.
My love.
Always.

TABLE OF CONTENTS

PART 3: POST-PARTUM

ACKNOWLEDGEMENTS

Becoming a mother opened up a whole new world to me. When I realized I was pregnant, there was really no way to know all the joy, tears, craziness, laughter, misery, frustration and fatigue that would ensue but as I was living through it, I thought that perhaps if someone had told me how they felt when they were pregnant or at home with a newborn, it might have helped me from thinking that I was nuts at times. It is true that I probably wouldn't have really absorbed what they were saying in the beginning but when I would have been in the thick of things, I would have found solace in the recollection that all of us have our challenges at some point or another when bringing a new life into the world.

For helping me overcome the challenges and for supporting me as I wrote this book, I gratefully thank:

My husband Ted. You still make me laugh after 23 years and despite never cooking, you somehow made sure I was eating those first weeks after I gave birth. A cherished memory is you physically putting forkfuls of food in my mouth as I was trying to figure out all this breastfeeding business. Our babies are not babies anymore but do you think you could try preparing a meal for me every once in awhile? It is definitely a turn on. Who knows, you might get lucky. No promises though.

My mom, for all the meals you prepared and popped in my freezer so that I would have one less thing to worry about, for coming to stay with us as much as possible so that you could give me a break from 24/7 baby, for teaching me your ways and for letting me teach you some of my ways.

My dad, for never doubting me and always encouraging me to "Keep going", for living without mom for weeks at a time so that she could come help me, and for crawling around on the floor to play with your grandchildren.

My mother-in-law, for taking care of me when I was pregnant with the stomach flu and had a toddler to boot. You saw me at my worst and you cared for me like I was your own child.

My father-in-law, for driving in the middle of the night to come care for my toddler when I went into labor despite your minor night-time driving anxieties, and for always making my children laugh with all your silly games.

My doctor, Oliver Nguan. Despite not being there for the birth of my first because your wife had the nerve to give birth a couple days before me or for my second because she was just in too much of a hurry to get out, you always offered sound medical advice and an opinion I could trust.

The doctors and nurses who helped to bring my daughters into this world, for knowing what you were doing, for not commenting on the sad state of affairs *down there* and for reminding my husband to snap some pictures during the birth.

The hospital cafeteria for putting together half-decent meals during my hospital stay.

My co-workers for listening to me bitch and moan about how miserable I was when I was pregnant.

All the moms out there who shared a horror-story or two about pregnancy and raising babies. Not the ones describing the medical horrors. Those I could have done without, thank you very much.

The Algonquin College School of Media & Design and specifically, Sundus Asif, for your creative ideas and the beautiful cover you created for this book.

My friends for giving me your thoughts, suggestions and encouragement as I slowly pieced together this book.

Those who have followed my blog and encouraged me to continue writing.

All the people who repeatedly asked *"Did you finish your book yet?"* It kept me from quitting even though I wanted to wring your necks on occasion.

And finally, I would like to thank my two daughters, Eva and Gia, for teaching me how to love unconditionally. You make mommy crazy sometimes but I hope you realize the sheer joy you bring into this world and what an adventure it has been from the first moment I knew you were coming. All I want is for you to feel loved and safe. Now get to bed already!

FROM THE AUTHOR

As I squatted awkwardly in the office bathroom back in early 2004, peeing on the stick, I just knew I was pregnant. I could feel it. Yes. There it was. That little '+' sign. I was ecstatic, my heart started racing and I couldn't wait to get started on the journey. It was going to be a glorious time. And it was, for about a month. And then the misery began. *"What did I get myself into?" "Why aren't I the happiest woman in the world?" "What is wrong with me?"* I am not a doctor nor a nurse nor a healthcare professional of any sort. I am however a mother, a mom, Mommy and I want to say that I hated being pregnant. Did it twice, and hated it twice.

When I was pregnant with my first child, I read a few books on what to expect during my pregnancy, what to expect after the birth, and what to expect the first year. It was hard to keep focused because there was so much information. I love to read but this felt like homework. These pregnancy books were massive. Where was the book that would prepare me for pregnancy and raising babies, help me understand what it was going to feel like, and that I could get absorbed in as if I was reading a novel?

I read about the moment by moment progress of this baby growing inside of me, the physical changes occurring in my body, and all the possible complications (which scared the crap out of me by the way), but what about how I was feeling? Everything I was reading or watching was preparing me for the physical aspects of a growing baby, for giving birth to a baby, and for the material things I would have to buy to care for this baby, but nothing was preparing me for the emotional ups and downs associated with pregnancy and raising this child. Why wasn't anyone describing what really happens during childbirth or the initial pain of breastfeeding? Why wasn't anyone warning me that I may one day find myself in the fetal position begging for my baby's crying to stop and that it would be perfectly normal?

I wish someone would have given me a more realistic view so that I wouldn't have felt so alone. Pregnancy and raising a baby isn't just fashion and beautiful nurseries nor is it just clinical details. It is an amazing experience, rewarding, fun and also extremely hard, painful, and sometimes scary as hell.

As for me, I hated being pregnant. It's ok to hate it. It doesn't however mean that you will love your baby any less so don't worry if you're feeling miserable. Your life will change forever now that you are having a baby. Some of those changes will be good, some bad and some really ugly. For now, while that baby is still tucked in your belly, put up your feet (if only for a few minutes at a time) and read on to learn some, cringe some and hopefully giggle a lot.

By the way, I would love to hear about your pregnancy and child rearing adventures. Looking forward to hearing from you at *babynowwhat-feedback@yahoo.ca*.

Congratulations! Get ready for the ride.

Katina

PART 1

PREGNANCY

CHAPTER 1

OH MY GOODNESS, HERE WE GO!

That was my first thought when I saw that little '+' sign. We had just started trying to have a baby, my period was a few days late and I had the brilliant idea while at work to walk over to the drugstore and pick up a pregnancy test. I couldn't wait to find out for sure so I squeezed myself into the bathroom stall, hiked up my skirt, did my business and then waited. Those few minutes waiting for the result seemed like forever and suddenly my heart was racing and a great wave of relief overtook me. *"Phew!"* I was actually capable of getting pregnant. My body worked. We did it. *"Now what?"*

In that instant, all the focus shifted to my belly and the baby that was growing inside of me. It was going to be an amazing nine months. My skin would glow, I would have the perfect pregnant belly, look fabulous in all the latest maternity wear and the nursery would look like it was straight out of the pages of a magazine.

When my husband and I were thinking of starting our family, it seemed that we heard so many stories of people struggling to have a baby and of the obstacles that these couples faced in trying to expand their families. Subconsciously, that was my biggest concern at the time. Will we have any issues getting pregnant? What if something is wrong? You always assume that you can have babies. It's natural, right? But how do you really know what's going on inside your body? I guess I'm just a worrier by nature but I'll admit that I let out a big sigh of relief when the test came back positive. Done, pregnant, the rest would be just fine. I never really thought about what I was about to embark on safe for the acceptance that it was going to be a lot of work and we were at the stage in our lives and relationship where we were ready to take it on.

Who would have thought that only a few short weeks into my pregnancy, I would feel trapped in my own body? All these things were happening to me, both physically and emotionally and I didn't know what to do about it.

In our celebrity-obsessed world, we are constantly bombarded with what celebrities have to say about their pregnancies. My brain would zero in on all these women telling me how they loved being pregnant, how it was an amazing experience. I remember reading a headline on one of those entertainment magazines quoting a famous actress that said she would love to be pregnant forever. The mere thought of a *forever* pregnancy makes me want to throw up. Even today.

It wasn't just the celebrities that were going on and on about how they loved pregnancy, it seemed like it was every pregnant woman I spoke with. Since that time, I have met other women who endured pregnancy in the same way I did but back then it seemed everyone I spoke with loved it. Mind you, these same women shared with me quite a few childbirth horror stories but the general consensus was that pregnancy was fantastic. Needless to say, they would look at me in shock when I bluntly proclaimed my hatred for it. *"How can they love being pregnant? I'm miserable."*

CHAPTER 2

HELLO NAUSEA

Everyone knows that for us humans, pregnancy is a nine month process. However, when you are pregnant, you immediately start speaking in terms of *weeks*. A typical pregnancy is 40-weeks and you begin counting from the first day of your last period. That is how you or your doctor can estimate your due date. And to all those women who claim they were pregnant for 10 months, unless you gave birth significantly past your due date, you are wrong. Do the math.

So let me explain a little bit of what my pregnancy was like. For the first few weeks, I would put my hand on my belly every once in a while but that was about it. I'm not quite sure what I was expecting to feel by doing this. You see, despite being excited, I didn't feel any different physically. Except that I had missed a period which in and of itself is a pretty sweet deal. In any case, I craved to feel different because it still didn't seem real to me. *"I'm pregnant? Really? How do you know?"*

At the six week mark of my pregnancy, my husband and I still had not shared the news with anyone, just keeping it to ourselves for a little bit longer not for any superstitious reasons (at least I don't think so) but more to have it be our personal secret. We were in the car with my brother and sister-in-law, driving to a restaurant, and we were doing our typical routine of talking about the food, what we would order, how hungry we were, and working ourselves up into a frenzy on our way there. Then my brother suggested steak. The sweating began, my stomach turned upside down and I was having trouble breathing. I instantly wanted to throw up. As I rolled down my window to get some air, my sister-in-law said *"What's wrong?"* *"Nothing"* I said, *"just a little hot"*. She looked me right in the eyes, smiled, and screamed *"You're pregnant!"*

I should mention that she was a few months pregnant with her first child and once you are pregnant, you acquire some kind of cosmic power that allows you to sense all the subtle clues and with relative ease pick out all the *in-the-closet* pregnant women out there.

Everyone was happy, congratulations all around, great. All I could picture was a raw steak on a plate staring at me. *"Hello nausea, nice to meet you, can you stick around for awhile so we can really get to know each other?"*

And so it began. There was no turning back now. One second I felt perfectly fine, the next I had morning sickness. This was definitely not the pregnancy feeling that I was craving. It really was that sudden. Although referred to as morning sickness, what I experienced was all day, everyday sickness. The doctor suggested I take only half the pre-natal vitamin instead of that horse-sized pill I was gagging down every morning, to eat smaller meals, to snack throughout the day and avoid fatty foods. He even prescribed anti-nausea medication. Friends suggested I drink ginger tea. I tried it all. Nothing worked.

I would throw up almost immediately after eating but the feeling of nausea never subsided. In my opinion, of all the *not-really-so-bad-in-the-grand-scheme-of-things* that a person can suffer from, nausea is the worst. I hate nausea.

As painful and as miserable as I felt, I also felt sorry for my husband. He just looked lost not knowing what to do to help and as so often happens with men when they don't know what to do, they start barking out orders. The most memorable refrain went a little bit like this, *"Stop throwing up. Just stop. Stop it. STOP!!"* as I was heaving into the toilet. *"Really helpful honey, thanks."* You know what? If I'm being honest, I didn't feel sorry for him. I probably didn't even give one second of thought to how he was feeling. I was too busy puking all the time. Forgive me for not being able to multi-task.

Well I finally did stop throwing up after six months but by the time the nausea went away, I was heading into my final trimester with its own slew of issues.

In case you were wondering about my second pregnancy and how that went I am happy to report that it was much better. Oh wait, no it wasn't, I just blocked it out. Maybe it's some sort of post-traumatic stress thing. The second time around, I didn't bother taking the anti-nausea medication my doctor recommended since I didn't particularly feel they made a difference in my first pregnancy. For some women, these pills do help though, particularly if you are so nauseous that you cannot eat anything and are not gaining sufficient weight so make sure you discuss with your doctor to determine what the right course of action is. In my case, lack of weight gain was never really a concern.

Before I move on, it is important to mention that not all women experience nausea and vomiting with their pregnancies or if they do, maybe not to this extreme. This is completely normal and I really do not think that you can tell one way or another whether you will experience these symptoms. If however you were, or are, one of the women without nausea during pregnancy, I hate you. Okay, I said it, now let's move on.

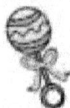

CHAPTER 3

WHAT IS THAT SMELL?

For some people, pregnancy brings with it heightened senses, aversion to certain foods and/or cravings for other foods. I fully expected to have cravings, it was hardwired in my brain that all pregnant women have them, but with my first pregnancy there were no intense cravings for anything. With the onset of nausea however, my sense of smell went through the roof and that is something I didn't anticipate in the least. My nostrils were constantly being bombarded by all the odors out there and I often found the smells to be overwhelming. Many smells were potent but at least tolerable while others were completely unbearable and would have me heaving in an instant.

I have since heard of pregnant women who suddenly find themselves disgusted at random things like the smell of coffee, the smell of food or even the smell of their own partner. For both of my pregnancies, the smell of leather would instantly make me gag. My leather blazer as well as our couch had an odor with skunk-like intensity. Needless to say, I stopped wearing that blazer while pregnant. As a matter of fact I've never worn it since. It was really nice. *"Where did I hide it?"*

Under the best of circumstances, I pee often. Ask anyone who knows me. However, even for my high standards of what constitutes normal, the frequency of times I would have to *go* during pregnancy was ridiculous. I often felt that half my day was spent in the washroom, particularly in my first and last trimesters. During the workday, if you wanted to chat, you were practically guaranteed to find me in the washroom. If I wasn't throwing up, I was peeing. Or both. You get the picture. An added bonus was that where I worked, the washrooms were equipped with a motion-detecting air freshener that would annoyingly *spritz* every time I walked in so that even if I was only heading in there to pee, that Lily of the Valley smell would guarantee me at least some minor retching.

Above all other smells however was the smell of garlic powder. That blasted garlic powder. I knew there was a smell in my kitchen that I could not stand. For days I could not figure out what it was when finally, unable to tolerate it anymore, I began sniffing inside the kitchen cabinets like a bloodhound until I reached the spice rack. The concentrated smell in that little jar of garlic powder brought me to my knees it was so overwhelming.

To this day, I still get *flashback queasiness* (I coined the term, feel free to use it) when I smell any of these items. It is highly probable that these particular smells may have no effect on you however don't be surprised if you do find that you develop super-hero senses during your pregnancy.

As for cravings, I only had them with my second pregnancy but there were quite a few of them. For some women, the cravings can seem somewhat bizarre and appear almost out of nowhere. At first I didn't even realize that I was having cravings but then suddenly I was drinking iced Tea everyday and guzzling down mineral water all the time, both of which I never drank before and drink only occasionally ever since. I also had a peculiar craving to chew on crushed ice. All the time. Maybe it was because it helped with the nausea but try figuring out how to get your hands on ice during the workday. I will give a shout out to Starbucks™ because they were the ones that saved me. At first I would order something to eat and ask them for a glass of ice water. Eventually, after one too many sweets, I confessed to the barista *"I'm pregnant and I know this sounds weird but could you just please give me a cup of ice?"*.

CHAPTER 4

I'M QUITTING!

Pregnancy books warn that you may experience some fatigue and sleepiness in the first months of pregnancy but most of us, already busy with our day to day lives, gloss over those words and think *"Yeah, whatever, I've been tired before"*. We were wrong. Perhaps we were tired after some nights of partying and heading straight to school or work afterwards, but that was for a day, maybe two, tops. During the first trimester, many women experience life-draining fatigue. Combine this with the feeling of nausea and getting out of bed each morning requires super-human strength and staying awake all day becomes virtually impossible.

During that time, there was not a morning that I did not wake up and contemplate quitting my job. Being a high energy individual working in a high-paced sales environment made this stage of pregnancy extremely painful. Sitting through presentations felt like putting needles in my eyes. Clients would be speaking with me and my mind was drifting. *"Do you think they will notice if I close my eyes for a second?"*

Like many of us in the workforce today know, open concept offices are not conducive to sneaking in rest time during the work day without anyone noticing. *"How can someone get a little bit of shut eye during the day?"* In my case, I would conjure up some important customer call that needed to be made privately and head off to find a boardroom, close the door, sit down, put up my feet and just close my eyes for a few minutes. Luckily I was never caught. A female co-worker, who was pregnant around the same time, confessed that some days, between sales calls, she would pull her car over, park, and take a quick nap in the car. This was completely understandable to me but many others would scoff at her laziness. By the time I would get home each day, there was absolutely no gas left in my tank and I would plop down on the sofa drained.

At least this time doesn't last too long however it is a rough period, particularly if you haven't yet told people that you are pregnant. People inevitably start gossiping *"What's wrong with her? She's acting weird. I bet you she's pregnant."* The second time around I told everyone straight out. No need to try and hide what I was going through right? *"Hey everybody, if I look sick, or tired, or act weird, it's because I'm pregnant! Deal with it because I have enough shit to deal with."*

CHAPTER 5

BURN BABY BURN

There are so many things that you have to deal with both emotionally and physically throughout your pregnancy. *"Am I ready for this?"*, *"Is my baby growing normally?"*, *"Do I look fat?"*, *"Will I be a good mother?"* As if all that wasn't enough, the last thing that I needed to be worrying about was that I was turning into my father, the king of heartburn. Heartburn and indigestion became a painful part of everyday life and fruit-flavoured antacids were my new best friend. I popped those bad boys like they were candies. They were everywhere, in the medicine cabinet, on my nightstand, at work. I'm sure I could probably still dig up some of that powdery residue out of the bottom of my purse.

Second to nausea, heartburn was the most painful part of both my pregnancies. It also seemed like every time someone would see how uncomfortable I was they would undoubtedly proclaim that heartburn during pregnancy meant that the baby would be born with lots of hair. *"Great! I'm sure she'll be born with pigtails."*

With both pregnancies, I felt that gut wrenching burn until the exact second the baby was born. The relief was immediate when that pressure was gone. Finally I could breathe again. By the way, both girls were in fact born with a full head of hair but at least nothing frighteningly wolf-like.

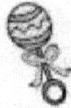

CHAPTER 6

PLEASE STEP ON THE SCALE

Throughout your pregnancy, your doctor will want to see you on a regular basis. At first it will be monthly, then biweekly and then weekly until you deliver. I hope you have an understanding employer or a doctor with flexible hours to make scheduling easier. Your appointments will vary; you will most certainly have blood tests done to screen for a number of items including hepatitis and HIV (*"Honey this better come back negative or we'll have bigger problems to deal with"*), your doctor will measure the size of your belly, take your blood pressure, and take a urine sample to analyse for protein levels on a regular basis and, from time to time, you will be able to listen to the baby's heartbeat and be examined in all those unmentionable places.

If a good old pelvic exam isn't enough for you, around week 36, your doctor may also conduct a test to see whether you are a Group B strep carrier (it's a type of bacteria). From a health perspective, being a carrier is not necessarily a big deal for the expectant mom however it could pose an infection risk for the baby during childbirth so it is important to know in advance in order to take precautionary measures. Sounds simple enough when the doctor explains this to you but the test involves a rectal swab. I repeat, a rectal swab. *"Come on! Aren't things awkward enough?"* The test takes a fraction of a second and some of you may not care at all, but I was a sweaty mess not knowing what to expect. And men worry about prostate exams! They have no clue the embarrassing things women endure in a doctor's office.

Speaking of embarrassing things, the one certainty at every doctor's appointment is the weigh-in. While I understand the clinical requirement for this, to ensure that the baby is not growing at some unreasonable rate, or conversely, not growing enough, I do not know if there is a pregnant woman out there, even the 9-month pregnant *skinnies* who somehow look like all they have is a bit of water retention, who likes the weigh-in. I put on 44lbs and 40lbs respectively for my two pregnancies; nothing too unreasonable although I admit that some of the pregnancy pictures were highly unflattering. There is no denying that I was big, but in no way was I ridiculously huge. Nevertheless, I always felt like a cow getting on that scale. The nurse and doctor would have a slight little smirk on their faces when I would step on the scale. And you know what they are thinking, don't you?*"Three pounds in one week. Wow."*

My only thought on the weight issue is not to let it become the focus of your pregnancy. You are creating a life inside of you. Focus on being strong and healthy, both physically and emotionally. We have all heard of women who fear that pregnancy will ruin their bodies and either avoid getting pregnant altogether or restrict their calories throughout their pregnancy. I'm fairly certain that's not a good thing.

In Canada, your doctor will typically schedule an ultrasound at the 12- and 20-week mark of your pregnancy. Pregnancy ultrasounds are exciting because you are able to see your baby on the monitor, maybe even doing a few somersaults, however the technologist will be taking measurements of your baby and assessing any potential abnormalities, so don't be surprised if you find yourself feeling stressed during the procedure. At the 20-week ultrasound it may be possible to determine your baby's gender depending on whether your baby chooses to cooperate and show off a bit. My two cents on whether to find out the sex of your baby or whether to wait is to say that I loved finding out early. Knowing what I was having connected me with my baby and it most definitely made the whole pregnancy more real for my husband. And who says it's not a surprise? It is a surprise; the surprise just comes at 20 weeks rather than at 40 weeks. We asked the technician to write down the baby's gender on a piece of paper which we then opened by ourselves in private. Thanks to my friend Jen for suggesting we do this. It was a great idea. My husband still carries that little piece of paper in his wallet and it can instantaneously bring back all the emotions we felt the moment we first read the word *GIRL*.

A final note on the ultrasound; you have to drink a lot of water prior to the procedure in a short period of time. By *a lot* I mean a ridiculous amount of water (6-8 glasses). This fills you up with fluid and makes it easier for the technician to get a good look at the baby but when you are nauseous from pregnancy to begin with, it seems impossible to get all that water down. When they called me in to the examination room, I lay reclined on the bed, with the cold ultrasound jelly on my stomach, and I was so nervous and excited that I was about to see my baby for the first time. By this time though, the water had made its way through my system and I was struggling not to scream at the technician to hurry up. Slight panic attack for sure but seeing the look on my husband's face when he saw our baby on the monitor made it all worth it. And then I took the longest pee of my life.

CHAPTER 7

WHAT IS HAPPENING TO ME?

The human body is fascinating and weird but usually, by the time a woman gets pregnant, she is pretty familiar with her own body, how it looks, how it feels and how it works. Pregnancy shakes everything up quite a bit as your body changes right in front of your eyes in many more ways than the obvious belly thing.

On a purely superficial level, the one cool thing about pregnancy was my hair. For those who don't know me, I have long thick hair under normal circumstances so it's not as if pregnancy is a hair miracle however I did get significantly more compliments about my hair during my pregnancy than at any other time. Maybe it was the only thing they could think of complimenting but it just seemed to be extra thick and extra shiny all the time and grew at an almost alarming rate. This meant that there was so much more hair to shed once the baby was born. That's right, you'll see.

My perky B-cup breasts also started to change during pregnancy. They started to feel fuller, heavier and the areolas got slightly darker. You might even begin to see a network of bluish lines appear under the skin of your breasts and across your chest as the blood supply to the breasts increases. For me, pregnancy boobs were big and fun. Breast changes were more pronounced and traumatic after giving birth so we will re-visit this subject later but I will note that two breastfed children later, I am now an only-slightly-less perky B-cup. But it did take quite some time to get there. For a long time after breastfeeding, my breasts looked normal enough but they didn't feel the same. The texture of the breast tissue had changed and I can only describe it as a feeling of emptiness. They were just too soft. The combination of pregnancy and breastfeeding can really mess things up and you may find you have smaller or droopy breasts after all is said and done which can be very hard on the self-esteem. I don't think there is any way to know what the outcome will be but make sure you wear appropriate bras with the right amount of support to try and minimize the sag factor.

As for your belly, it will get big. Maybe not blimp size, but big enough that you will not feel like the same person anymore. In your first trimester (weeks 1 – 13), it will probably just feel like a tightening in your lower abdomen, almost as if you have a rock right above your pubic bone. After a few weeks you will start to feel thicker (what an ugly word) around the waist but if anyone even notices the change they will think that perhaps you have been indulging in a few too many desserts.

By the second trimester (weeks 14 to 27), your belly will slowly start to get bigger as your baby grows. There are so many different shapes of pregnant bellies out there. For both my pregnancies, my belly was big and round and would swell out from right under my breasts. It almost felt as if I was pregnant all around my torso, not just in the front. Other women have very low bellies where it seems that all the action is taking place between the belly button and the pubic area. You can't even tell they are pregnant when they have their back to you.

At the latter stages of my pregnancy, my belly was so high that I had to put my hand on my belly, right under my breasts, and push down a little bit because I felt I could not breathe. The doctors say that the belly was pushing against my diaphragm so I couldn't fully expand my lungs but it did make for very shallow breaths and a fairly high resting heart rate.

All in all, it is freaky to watch your belly grow throughout the nine months. In the last trimester (weeks 28 – 40), when the baby is crammed in there and your skin has been stretched so taut, you will quite literally be able to see the outline of your baby under your belly. Remember the television mini-series "V" from the 80's where the alien head grew right out of the woman's belly? Probably not but that's what it reminded me of. There will be times where you may be able to make out the outline of a foot, or hand, or head pushing up against your skin.

With all this belly and breast growth, your skin is constantly stretching. If you haven't noticed already, you will soon realize that a lot of women are obsessed with the prevention of stretch marks during their pregnancies. You might be one of them. The marketing machine works overtime in promoting the many miracle creams to pregnant women, and perhaps they work for some, but just remember that sometimes, no matter what you do, stretch marks will appear.

In my case, I thought I was in the clear. I wasn't too vigilante with the creams during my pregnancy because I found them either too smelly (which made me nauseous) or too oily (which stained my clothes). Although both my belly and my breasts were extremely itchy throughout my pregnancy, I did not see any hint of a stretch mark. Then I gave birth and my belly started to shrink. As I slowly got my pre-pregnancy figure back I noticed stretch marks appearing. There weren't many, but they were definitely there. *"Shit! Why now? My belly is not stretching anymore."* So why do they call them stretch marks? I was fooled. Consider yourselves warned: Pregnancy may lead to stretch marks and shrink marks. They will fade over time but these battle scars will never disappear.

Apparently people have a faint white line down the centre of their abdomen to the top of the pubic bone which is called the *linea alba*. I had never noticed this before and I still can't see it to this day. Maybe I'm just too pale. During pregnancy, because of all those hormone changes, some people, like me, get a darkening of that line, thus it is renamed the *linea nigra*, or black line. It looks kind of like you traced a line vertically down your belly with a black marker and then tried to wash it off. It is faded but still there. If you can't quite visualize what I am talking about, over the next few years you will become very familiar with the *faded-marker* look as your child gets older and becomes fascinated with drawing on anything in site and you painstakingly try to wash off marker stains from your lovely sofa.

As for the *linea nigra*, no big deal, it goes away but it looks weird for a while all the same. Funny how you never see the linea nigra in those beautiful magazine pictures of pregnant women in bikinis. I guess it must have been airbrushed out along with the cellulite and stretch marks.

An important symptom to not ignore during your pregnancy is sensitivity to the sun. During my second pregnancy, while on holidays and fully lathered up with a high SPF sunscreen, my skin was still tanning. The tan eventually faded however I did get permanent darkening on certain parts of my face. Concealer has always been part of my daily makeup routine but now it's not only for my dark under-eye circles. I have seen this happen to several friends so take extra care when you are out in the sun.

CHAPTER 8

CLOSE YOUR EYES

Except for some angst-filled nights during university, I never had any sleep problems prior to becoming pregnant. With my first pregnancy, there was physical discomfort which led to the occasional sleepless night but with my second, it was extreme insomnia. Pregnancy transformed me into a wandering night creature, roaming from room to room, desperately trying to get comfortable. Stomach sleeping was obviously a no-no so I would spend the first few hours of the night in bed flipping from side to side. By the way, you can't sleep on your back during pregnancy because your growing belly places too much weight on your back and all your internal organs which can cause problems with breathing and circulation. I was too hot with the comforter so I would kick it off but then I got too cold so I would cover myself. Then I would stick my feet out because they were too hot all the while driving my husband crazy. Now that I think about it, it was probably all his fault – that man is a freaking furnace.

Inevitably I would get up and head to the guest room where I would toss and turn for a while. Then I would head to the living room and have a snack or read or watch a movie. Needless to say, it was stressful when we had company sleeping over because my nightly roaming around the house in my various states of undress was hindered. I didn't want to disturb anyone else's sleep but more importantly, I didn't want anyone to see me slamming back a sandwich at three in the morning.

Most nights would end with me on the sofa and my body eventually shutting down around four or five in the morning just in time for the alarm to ring in the start of a brand new day. With my second pregnancy, these sleepless nights got me ready for what lay ahead once the baby was born. In fact I had significantly more energy once the baby came because the physical discomfort was gone thus I was able to get much more sleep than during pregnancy.

Be aware that this extra energy bonus was definitely only with my second child. With my first, I thought I was going to die of fatigue in the weeks after her birth and I was begging to sleep for just one more minute. Time doesn't make you forget how hard it is. It has been eight years and I still remember my baby crying in the middle of night as I lay on my bed in the fetal position, crying, in my milk-stained T-shirt. I'm getting ahead of myself though.

CHAPTER 9

YOU GIVE ME FEVER

Let me describe a little scenario that many women are familiar with. You and your partner are sitting in the car, driving around, running errands perhaps or, better yet, going out for a romantic dinner. Everything is just great when suddenly you are arguing over the thermostat. He says *"It's too hot in here"*, you say *"I'm freezing"*. And back and forth it goes. Men rarely complain that they are cold; women always seem to have cold hands. As I'm typing this now, my hands are practically ice cubes.

When pregnant however, you may find that your internal thermostat changes. I was on fire most of the time and that lasted for well over a year after giving birth. My menstrual cycle didn't start up again until about 8 months post-partum so I would joke that I was getting a taste of what menopause would be like with the unexpected hot flashes, night sweats, all that sexy stuff.

Not all moms experience overheating and perhaps it might have been amplified due to the time of the year that I was pregnant. With both children, I was *big* pregnant throughout the summer months which probably pushed my heat meter up higher but I do have one hilarious anecdote that I will share if for no other reason than to make fun of my brother a little bit.

As I mentioned earlier, my sister-in-law was pregnant at the same time as I was and gave birth to her son in late August. My husband and I were visiting from out of town just days before she gave birth. We were in the midst of a heat wave so between the two pregnant women there were quite the lovely swollen ankles on full display and the air conditioner was cranked up really high. The four of us were sitting at the kitchen table, chatting about random things when my brother shivered. He kept on speaking but slowly got up and started walking towards the thermostat. Suddenly we were witnessing something straight out of a horror movie. With an almost demonic timbre to her voice my sister-in-law warned him that if he so much as put a finger on that thermostat, she would kill him. Big macho brother quickly stepped away from the thermostat in fear. I laughed so hard I almost wet my pants.

CHAPTER 10

BABY BRAIN

Let me give you a little insight into the type of person I am. First generation Canadian, daughter of Greek immigrants, youngest of three children, only daughter. My parents worked from the time they landed in Canada which meant I would have to wake myself for school each day, get dressed, do homework by myself, help translate any letters my parents couldn't understand, and basically help with household responsibilities.

I was a straight 'A' student, perfectionist, graduated with honours from university and went on to get a Masters degree in Mathematics. My husband and I met on the first day of college, sparks flew, and we've been together ever since. I work hard, I can hold my own in any discussion, multitask like the best of them, and pride myself on being a pretty smart cookie. Blah, blah, blah. My point is, what the hell happened to me during pregnancy? I turned into a bumbling idiot. I'm exaggerating a bit but during pregnancy you may feel that you are losing more and more brain cells each day. I often walked around feeling like my brain was foggy and I had difficulty remembering from one minute to the next what I was looking for or where I was going. And I wasn't just imagining this. My husband noticed and casually mentioned that he was *"sort of, kind of, liking my dumb period"*.

This period however was disconcerting for me; it just felt weird knowing that no matter how much I tried to concentrate or remember something, it was all too fuzzy up there. I'm not sure it really went away. About a year after the birth of my second child, I spoke with my doctor and asked why, from time to time, I still had difficulty concentrating and remembering things. Based on my symptoms, he immediately suspected low iron and sent me for blood work.

It turns out that women in general have a difficult time maintaining normal iron levels because of the blood loss experienced monthly due to menstruation but this can be even more challenging after having babies. For many women, post-pregnancy menstrual flow can be much heavier than before and already low iron stores can get depleted rather quickly. These days, I can tell with relative ease if my iron level is getting low because I start getting headaches and that fuzzy brain feeling returns. I try to eat properly, take an iron supplement as required and I've gotten really good at making lists and writing things down so I don't forget.

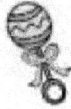

CHAPTER 11

PLAN? WHAT PLAN?

The closer you get to the end of your pregnancy, the more anxious you will probably begin to feel as you question whether you are ready. There are so many unknowns with giving birth that it can feel overwhelming. In general, I was relatively calm since I was too busy either dealing with my physical discomfort or with work to let my mind wander to the fact that in a few short weeks a birth would be taking place and I would be in the lead role. Every so often though, my heart would start racing unexpectedly, my legs would turn to jelly and I would think *"Holy shit! I'm going to have a baby!!"*

I imagine that most experts would suggest that being as informed as possible and making a plan helps reduce any anxiety. So that's what so many pregnant women do. They plan, they prepare for the unexpected so that they feel in control of the situation. I would speak with others who have already gone through this, asked questions, read books, signed up for pre-natal classes, and prepared a birthing plan, all with the intent of learning everything I possibly could about what was coming and ensuring that everyone knew what type of delivery I wanted. Let's cut to the chase however. The most worrisome part for the uninitiated is the actual *birthing* process. *"How will I know that I'm in labor? When should I go to the hospital? How much will it hurt? Epidural or not?"*

Pre-natal classes promised to educate my husband and I on what labor would be like and how to care for our newborn. They provided us the opportunity to spend some time with other couples who were going through similar life events as well as giving us a feel for where to go when the day finally arrived. They were however completely off the mark from the labor reality I experienced.

During one of the classes, we were watching a movie that looked like it was filmed back in the 70's with the narrator explaining the onset of labor and suggesting we not rush to the hospital immediately. The soothing voice suggests you go for a walk with your husband instead or perhaps bake a cake to pass the time and reminds you that the cake will be a pleasant treat when you return from the hospital. I thought this was priceless and struggled not to laugh out loud in class. *"You have got to be kidding me! Bake a cake?!?!"* Needless to say, I didn't jot that suggestion down on my To Do List. My husband recalls another suggestion to go watch a movie at the onset of labor. Again, didn't make the list.

Other suggestions included bringing items to the hospital such as music, candles or massage oils to help soothe you during labor. Having experienced labor and delivery twice, I honestly can't imagine arriving at the hospital in the midst of contractions and even remembering to take these items out of my bag.

There was way too much time devoted to breathing techniques which, in my opinion, makes you more anxious because unless you are in labor, breathing in this manner seems odd so you fear you won't remember how to do it properly when the time comes.

As for the birthing plan, some of the items that this plan typically outlines include where you want to have your baby, who you want present during the delivery, whether you would like pain medication, what measures doctors should take in order to deliver the baby and who will cut the umbilical cord. Samples of such birthing plans can easily be found online. That is where I found mine, filled it in and packed it early on in my little suitcase that I would be bringing with me to the hospital.

Upon arriving at the hospital however, my only focus was on handling the pain. At no point did I even remember that there was a birthing plan in my bag.

So here's my advice, based on no medical data whatsoever. First and foremost, listen to your doctor's advice throughout your pregnancy. Second, discuss any important birthing requests or instructions well in advance (eg. whether or not you will want pain medication). Third, when the time does come to have your baby

- Try and stay calm.

- Don't scream (it really doesn't help anyone).

- Monitor the time between any contractions.

- With each contraction, take deep breaths through your nose until the pain subsides. I did this with my second labor and it significantly helped with the pain and made me feel much less frantic than the first time. You can stop rolling your eyes now. It really did work. But who knows? Maybe something else will work for you. The goal however is to find something that calms you.

Finally, the most important thing I can stress is that once you do decide to get to the hospital (or whichever location you have chosen for the birth), stop trying to control the situation. The objective is to have a healthy, safe delivery so listen to the experts. The doctors and nurses know everything you need to know. They will tell you where to go, what to do, how to breathe, and when to push. Remember though that in the end, labor and delivery may not go down exactly as you had envisioned it in your mind but it bears repeating, you are bringing a life into this world and the only true objective should be for you and your baby to be healthy and safe.

As for me, in retrospect, I would give birth any day versus being pregnant. What are a few hours of pain versus discomfort for nine whole months? Mind you I did eventually have an epidural with both deliveries but I found birth much easier to deal with. Be forewarned however, I may be in the minority with my thinking.

CHAPTER 12

DECISIONS, DECISIONS

There are so many different types of women in this world at different stages in their lives, with various personalities, cultural backgrounds, and different external influences such as where they live and what circle of friends they have. There are many things that will influence what type of mother you will become, or at least plan on becoming.

For some women, there is somewhat of a denial that takes place with pregnancy. These women don't want to talk too much about what's going to happen, don't want to over think anything, don't prepare for the pending arrival, and appear to be somewhat clueless. Grandma usually needs to come to the rescue here.

For others, motherhood is such an organic process, there is a sense of comfort and ease with these women about everything that they are about to embark on. They are not uninformed but almost Zen about everything.

Finally there are the over-achievers. From my experience, the vast majority of women today fall into this final category. These are women who have lots of people around them who have gone through pregnancies and have a ton of suggestions to make, these women are very comfortable with the internet, research everything and want to make everything absolutely perfect.

There are many decisions that you will need to make when you are pregnant and I can safely say with a high degree of certainty that some women are not allowing themselves the opportunity to make decisions that will work best for them rather than succumbing to societal pressures of what they must do. *"Why do we make things so hard for ourselves?"*

Some of the hotly debated decisions that you will be faced with include:

• **Natural or Epidural?** I do not understand why this question can be so polarizing amongst women. In my opinion, why would I not want to take something to help ease some of the pain of childbirth? In fact, I don't even understand the use of the term *natural*. Why isn't childbirth with epidural considered natural? The baby is still making the same trip out of my body but I don't feel it as much and the doctors and nurses can do what they need to, when they need do, without worrying about me. I have read many arguments for and against the use of pain medication during childbirth but one person's experience doesn't necessarily mean that your experience will be the same. We do not live in a sterile world and there are plenty of toxins that are being transferred to your unborn baby because of the world we live in, the products we use and the food that most people consume. Weigh the risks and decide with those that are closest to you whether an epidural is the right chose for you. For those who prefer no medication, more power to you ladies, but let's all cut each other some slack and let people decide what feels right for them.

- **Breastfeeding or bottle?** Breastfeeding is the recommended form of feeding for babies because of scientific evidence demonstrating a long list of health, growth and development benefits for the newborn. The notion is so prevalent that I didn't even really think of another option and assumed that my baby would be born, I would put her on my breast, and nature would take its course. It unfortunately was not that simple but I would definitely say that once my baby and I got the hang of it, breastfeeding allowed for a great bonding experience and was a superbly convenient form of feeding with no worries about bottles, sterilizing equipment and warming up of formula. I will admit though that each time my child got sick with a cold I would think *"Didn't I read somewhere that all this breastfeeding was supposed to boost your immunity?"*

Breastfeeding however is not necessarily the right option for all new mothers and you should consider your situation before deciding (How long will you be off of work? Do you have other children to tend to? Was it a multiple birth? Do you feel uncomfortable with the idea of breastfeeding?). Once you decide, request that people respect your choice and if you change your mind again, that is your prerogative.

• **How long should I breastfeed?** Depending on where you live, there are different health guidelines for how long babies should be breastfed. The Canadian guideline that I followed indicated that babies should be breastfed exclusively for the first six months, and then continue to be breastfed along with solid foods for at least the first year of their life.

We followed this guideline fairly closely and I breastfed both my daughters exclusively for the first six months. They were both growing well according to their physician so there was no need to introduce other foods prior to six months. They were weaned off breast milk at approximately nine and eleven months respectively because it made sense. By this I mean, they bit me. In both cases, their razor sharp baby teeth suddenly chomped down on my nipple during a feeding one day and I was shocked by how painful it was. It didn't take long after that incident for the weaning process to begin. *"Hello bottle!"*

Some mothers however choose to breastfeed significantly longer. This is perfectly fine but my suggestion would be to ensure you are including the dads in the feeding process so they can also experience that bond with their baby and you don't start thinking they are useless.

If you do choose to continue breastfeeding longer, be aware that to the outside world it can look very bizarre to witness a *big* child asking for his mother's breast. Sitting in a coffee shop one morning, I witnessed a boy, who must have been about three years old, crying uncontrollably about something and then suddenly he climbed up into his mother's lap as she was talking with the boy's father. Without hesitation, he pulled up her shirt and popped her boob into his mouth. He only did this for a few seconds so my thought is that he was using his mother to pacify himself rather than for the nutritional benefits of breast milk but what do I know? It did seem odd however.

- **Pacifier or not?** Prior to getting pregnant I never thought that this was an issue since I assumed all babies have pacifiers. However, sources warned about potential issues when introducing the use of a pacifier or bottle to your baby because he or she may become confused with the different nipples and perhaps reject your breast for feedings. Sounds plausible right? Well it sure sounded plausible to me and I know it made me nervous. Another concern is the desire to teach your child to self-soothe so that they won't depend on the pacifier to calm down. *"Should I use a pacifier? Shouldn't I?"*

With my first, we quickly discovered that there were no issues and no confusion. Anything you put near her, she would pop in her mouth whether it was a pacifier, a breast, a bottle or a toy. *"Bring it on!"* This of course freaked me out as well because it seemed like she would never stop using her pacifier. She did stop though. They all do. So don't beat yourself up and let paranoia kick in when you look around and it feels like your baby is the only one with a pacifier.

Three years later, with my second who refused to take a pacifier, the tables had turned and I was praying for her to accept it when she was crying uncontrollably those first few months. At around the four- or five-month mark, she was alone with my husband one afternoon and he just popped it in her mouth when she was crying. Repeatedly. She gave up, realized she could soothe herself with this thing that her dad kept popping in her mouth. When she was calm, she just spit it back out. We were finally able to go out as a family and have some sense of security that if she started to lose it, there was something that could help us.

PART 2

LABOR

CHAPTER 13

IS THIS LABOR?

I should start by saying that I was extremely naïve about labor. Before my own pregnancy, I used to think that I would know labor was starting because my *water would break*. I always figured a gush of something would suddenly come out of me and off to the hospital I would go. That's how it was for my mother and for all my closest friends so I just assumed.

As I was reading about pregnancy and attending pre-natal classes, I learned however that this is not the most common onset for labor. Contractions are. I read about the signs of early labor which can include cramps, the baby descending into the pelvis, a change in your vaginal discharge, cervical dilation and increased frequency of Braxton-Hicks contractions. These practice contractions happen so that your body begins preparing itself for labor but they always have you second guessing whether they are the real thing. They mess with your mind.

I also learned that most first-time mothers go past their due date. *"Please don't let that happen to me!"* All of this just made determining the onset of labor more complicated. The closer I got to my due date the more I would think *"Was that a real contraction?"*, *"Is that gas or is that a contraction?"*, *"I'm feeling kind of moist down there. Is that what they mean by water breaking?"* These were a never-ending refrain in my brain.

After nine months of pregnancy, 39 weeks to be exact, I climbed into bed on a Wednesday night after a long day. I was absolutely exhausted and exhilarated as well because it had been a great day at work but I was now officially off on maternity leave. In typical fashion, I got up to go to the bathroom a short while later however this time, I saw blood on my underwear. Not a lot but enough that I thought to myself, *"Should I get this checked out?"* There wasn't any pain besides the usual pregnancy discomfort so I wasn't certain what to do. I chose to wait but first thing in the morning I went to the hospital where they gave me an ultrasound. The doctor checked me out, said that everything was fine and told me that I had at least another week before the baby would come. We were sent on our merry way and they casually mentioned that the baby looked big. Maybe a *10-pounder* was what was predicted. *"Great, thanks for that little tidbit of information."* I left the hospital and went shopping. At this point, I guess there was nothing I could do about it.

Having given birth twice, I will tell you that all the second-guessing about whether or not I was in labor was a complete waste of time and energy. Within a few short hours, not the week that had been predicted, when the baby did decide to come, I knew. No ifs, ands, or buts about it. I knew.

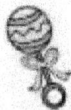

CHAPTER 14

TIME TO GO

It had been a long day spent in the hospital all morning and shopping in the afternoon. My husband and I had some dinner, watched some television then I decided to take a shower before bed. I finally climbed into bed at about 11 o'clock and began my now typical night time routine of flipping from side to side trying to get comfortable. Within minutes I felt this severe clenching in my belly. *"Holy shit! What was that?"* There really was no doubt what it was. It had to be a contraction. And so I did what any sane woman would do at that time, I checked the time (11:05pm) and then jumped out of bed to shave my legs and see what I could do to render my bikini area presentable. Quite honestly, I hadn't been able to see anything down there for quite some time so I had to pull out a mirror to see what state it was in.

11:20pm – Bam, another one.

Me: (excited) Wake up! It's time!

Husband: (all groggy) Time for what?

Me: (sarcastically) Time to party!

Husband: (confused) What?

Me: Get up you fool, I'm having the baby!!!

In pre-natal class they told us to wait, bake a cake, or go to the movies. What did we do? We got dressed, got our things together, and were out the door by midnight. I knew that this was not going to be a long drawn out labor. I could feel it in my bones. It was a twenty minute drive to the hospital and by the time I got there, my contractions were coming every 3 or 4 minutes. It was crazy.

As for contractions, you feel perfectly normal one second and then suddenly you feel an intense tightening in your abdomen. They do not feel like menstrual cramps as others have suggested. They are sharp, sudden, intensely strong and completely take your breath away. This of course had me clenching my face and holding my breath until the pain would subside but I do recommend you try and take deep breaths instead. I don't know what made me try this with my second pregnancy but it really helped. Squeezing somebody's hand at the same time really helped as well although warn them that they may lose sensation in their hand.

Besides all the craziness, I do remember that drive to the hospital very fondly. We called our families, told them we were on our way to have the baby, and then we drove quietly realizing that after fourteen years together, this would be the last time it would be just the two of us.

I was also scared to death because the words "10-pounder" were floating around in my brain. *"What did I get myself into?"*

CHAPTER 15

WHERE'S THE BATHROOM?

I struggled whether to include this section but it definitely was one of those things of pregnancy that nobody had warned me about so I do feel compelled to share. If we know each other, please never speak of this to me, pretend you never read this and I apologize for putting these images in your mind.

I walked slowly and painfully down that hospital corridor and got to the check-in desk (*"Is that what they call it?"*), told them I was in labor and then I waited for the nurses and doctors to determine whether they would let me stay or send me home to wait out the labor. I knew I wasn't going anywhere but I cooperated with their procedure and every couple of minutes, the wind would continue to get knocked out of me as another contraction would hit. My husband looked mortified as he quietly observed all of this. And then, with no warning whatsoever, the game I like to refer to as *contraction diarrhea* began.

In a blind panic, I darted down the corridor desperately looking for a bathroom and for the next half hour lost complete control of my bowels. That's right. Disgusting indeed. Lucky for me, it was a single washroom. Actually, lucky for everyone else. With every contraction, another wave of diarrhea would hit. Any pregnancy related constipation I suffered from was completely eradicated. I was a big disgusting mess, I desperately wanted this baby out of me, and I was still waiting for a nurse to check whether in fact my water had broken.

When this finally stopped, I pulled together any dignity that I had left, and walked back into the examining room to patiently wait for the nurse. Then, without warning, the floodgates burst open and in a flash, I was left sitting in a massive pool of fluid. No small trickle. Just one big whoosh. If I thought my husband looked mortified before he was now completely void of color. You know he was thinking *"What the *%!* is going on here?"*

The nurse walked in and thankfully was unfazed by what she saw, quickly checked to see how dilated I was which basically means she measured how much my cervix had opened. She proclaimed excitedly that I was already 6cm dilated (this is about 2.5 inches). Typically, pushing begins once you reach 10cm (about 4 inches) and for many women this process of dilation can be very long and tedious with only minor changes over long periods of time.

Things moved quickly for me however and at about 2:30am I was officially admitted to the hospital, changed into my hospital gown and was asked two things by the nurse.

First she asked whether I wanted an enema because many women poo during labor. *"What???? I didn't know that! Are you kidding me?"* By the way, take note that anybody who has children starts to use the word poo all the time. You'll see. My face turned red and I told her I didn't really expect to have any issues with that. She laughed and then thanked me. It's true, she thanked me. *"Poor lady, do you think the task of picking up labor-induced poo was in her job description?"*

Then she asked whether I wanted any pain medication. *"Yes indeed!"* I could barely breathe from the pain at this point.

One baby coming up!

CHAPTER 16

THIS IS A WORKOUT

The hospital staff gave me the green light to stay and then proceeded to get me set up comfortably in the delivery room. The anaesthesiologist showed up soon after and I didn't feel a thing when he gave me the epidural. He told me to lean forward; he worked gently on my lower back for a couple minutes, I felt a slight pick and that was it. Very shortly thereafter I started to feel the pain ease up. I could still feel the contractions but the medication had eased the pain significantly.

For those who haven't experienced this before, I'll create the visual. I was semi-reclined in a bed, no freaky stirrups or foot rests or anything like that. I had the epidural attached in my lower back, I had an IV attached to the top of my hand, and I had a baby monitor attached to my belly which was tracking the fetal heartbeat so you constantly hear this noise in the background and you know it's your baby. This machine also produces a graph so the hospital staff (and you) can clearly see the spikes when you are experiencing a contraction, how often they come, how evenly spaced they are. My husband loved this machine and every few minutes he would inform me that I was having another contraction. *"Uh, yeah, thanks for the scoop honey!"* Everyone was relaxed, monitoring all of this and waiting until I was dilated enough for pushing to begin. I was cracking jokes to pass the time which I tend to do when I'm nervous, my husband was resting on a recliner in the room sipping on a Gatorade (*"Seriously, don't get me started!!"*) and it seemed that everybody on staff at the hospital walked in at some point and got a view of my dilated cervix. At that point, I didn't care. *"Come one, come all!!"* But then, just like that, my contractions slowed down.

The doctor decided to induce contractions but that never really worked. Do you know why? Because they never turned the drip on! In any case, despite my weak, random contractions, I did manage to give birth to my daughter but boy did she make me work for it.

Pushing is timed to occur with each contraction. In other words, your body is naturally contracting in its attempt to expel this *foreign* object from inside and you push at the same time to help the baby vacate the premises quicker. By the way, I always thought *pushing* meant you force on your vagina, like when you pee but harder. Not at all. Pushing means you force yourself like you have to go number two. When your contractions are irregular or infrequent, the baby starts wandering back up to its old stomping ground and forgets that it was on its way out.

So I pushed in the traditional manner reclined in a bed (you know, like how you see on TV), I pushed while in a squat position hoping gravity would help, I pushed while on all fours because the nurses suggested it would help (and I felt like a complete fool in this position by the way) but in the end, I assumed the traditional position because I was tired and just wanted to lie down a bit. This lasted for close to four hours and I overheard the doctor tell the nurse that it was time to consider a C-section. *"What? Not a chance mister! After all this exertion there is no way I'm having a C-section!"* I bared down so hard I had that baby out in 20 minutes. She wasn't a 10-pounder as predicted but still a big 8 lb 6 ounces. There was some minor tearing which was stitched up but over the next 24 hours I began to feel like I had done the most intense workout of my life. I was obviously sore overall in my vaginal area but I had a hard time getting the hang of pushing properly and instead had been clenching my upper body. The next morning, my muscles were killing me. I was exhausted and would stay exhausted for months after this.

With my second child, it was practically a walk in the park. I say practically because let's be realistic, an 8lb child did take a trip down from my uterus through my vagina, no small feat, but I would wish such an easy labor for all women.

Labor started in an almost identical manner as with my first. I went to bed, woke up about an hour later to go to the bathroom and once again, I saw blood on my underwear. I called my in-laws who live about two hours away and asked them to drive down so they could stay with our daughter. We asked them to get ready and drive carefully, no need to rush but to get there as soon as they could. Within the hour, my contractions started and I sat on the sofa and waited, holding my 3-year old daughter's hand through each contraction. She was fantastic! My in-laws showed up about 3 hours after the initial call and by this point my contractions were roughly 2 minutes apart. No time for chit chat, we rushed out the door and headed to the hospital, got admitted right away, water broke, had just been administered the epidural and we were told by the nurses to get comfortable because this often takes awhile. *"Wrong!"*

Now you might be wondering why I chose to have the epidural since everything was moving so quickly. My thoughts are that if something should go wrong and they need to make a quick decision to perform a C-section for example, I wanted to be ready. But that's a personal decision and in the end, probably served no purpose with this delivery at all except to slightly numb the *ring of fire* effect as the baby crowned. This is the term my non-epidural using friend uses to describe the feeling of pain she experienced as her son was coming out.

Within minutes I felt nauseous. The nurse told me that it was the medication that was starting to take effect. As I was fidgeting in the bed in discomfort I somehow managed to move the baby monitor. There was no more signal and the nurse tried to fix things but couldn't find the heartbeat. Momentary panic and she asks if she can examine me internally. *"No need to ask lady! Check what needs to be checked!"* The nurse then lifted my gown and guess what was there? Yes, my baby was there. Not the whole thing, mind you, but the top of her head was there and the nurse screamed "Don't move, don't breathe, and don't push". Some random doctor came rushing in, smiled and told me to push once, push twice and that's it. Baby was born. No tearing, no stitches, no strain, nothing. I had a healthy baby and I felt like a million bucks.

As I held my brand new baby in my arms, doctors continued working down there, delivering the afterbirth. It's not something I was even aware was going on because I was too busy gazing into my baby's face however as my husband was snapping pictures of me and the baby, he managed to capture some lovely shots of the placenta in the background. Guess he wasn't aware of what was going on down there either.

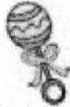

CHAPTER 17

STUFF I FORGOT TO MENTION

Before we move on, here are a few more tidbits that I wanted to highlight:

- Some women lose all sexual desire when they are pregnant while others are horny as hell. The same woman could feel a certain way with one pregnancy and completely different for the next. *"Who says that happened to me? I'm just saying."*

- Some women experience extreme leg discomfort, restlessness or painful cramping in their legs during pregnancy. This often happens while sleeping.

- Parking spots reserved for pregnant women are a beautiful thing. Some days, when finding a parking spot is proving to be somewhat of a challenge, I long to park in one of those reserved spots just to see if anyone says anything. *"How do you know whether I'm pregnant? Is there a rule that you have to be showing in order to use this spot?"*

- Some pregnant women glow while others struggle with skin problems such as acne. Some, like me, flip flop between the two extremes throughout the different stages of pregnancy. *"What happened to my face? Now I'm fat and ugly."*

- Many women are congested throughout their entire pregnancy. I went through boxes and boxes of tissues trying to rid myself of that stuffed up feeling.

- Some people just can't stop themselves from trying to predict the sex of your baby. Their theories rely on the shape of your belly, how you look or even by your mood. If you are huge, cranky and looking kind of ragged, people usually predict you're having a girl. *"Isn't that so sweet?"*

- The last couple of weeks before giving birth, you may walk around feeling like you have a bowling ball ready to fall out of your vagina. Things start getting pretty swollen down below.

- If having a vaginal birth, some doctors may perform an episiotomy which means they cut some tissue in order to enlarge the vaginal opening and facilitate the birth. Others choose to let any vaginal tearing occur naturally. Both require stitching.

- You will be wearing a pad for quite some time after having a vaginal birth since you will continue to bleed anywhere from a few days up to a couple of months. Some hospitals provide women with special pads during their stay. These pads are massive, starting from just under your belly button and wrapping around all the way up your bum. *"Could I feel any more unattractive?"* Once you are home, regular pads will do. By the way, *ixnay on the amponstay*. For those not versed in the art of Pig Latin, that means tampons are a no no.

- During your hospital stay, the nurse may pass by every so often to massage your belly, gently pushing in and down, squeezing out any potential blood clots. And you will feel the blood gushing out as she does this. You will also feel gushing blood when you sit or stand up from the bed. It's like you are one big juice box.

- The nurse may also want to check to see how the post-partum bleeding is coming along. This means that you will turn to your side and she will just peek right in there, monster pad and all. *"Did I mention that your dignity was tossed out along with your placenta?"*

- You will most likely have to take a sitz bath (i.e. sit in a tub or basin filled with warm water to cleanse and soothe your privates) or use a plastic bottle to squirt warm water on your privates for several days after the birth, particularly during urination to minimize the stinging sensation.

- You will be petrified to look at the damage down below after giving birth but you may be even more petrified to have your first bowel movement. At least I was. Hospitals will often provide women with a stool softener to get things all primed for that first post-partum poop. *"It's a medical term, abbreviation PPP, trust me."* I had given birth to a fairly large baby, through my vagina, and I was perhaps more nervous to go to the bathroom than I had been to give birth. It was no big deal when all was said and done but psychologically, it was pretty stressful. Everything felt like it was hanging on by a thread. *"Wait, I have stitches, everything is hanging on by a thread!"* I thought it was all just going to fall apart if I forced too much.

PART 3

POST-PARTUM

CHAPTER 18

THE FIRST DAYS

The first few days after giving birth are an absolute blur. The day gives way to night without you noticing, nurses are coming and going, things are quiet for prolonged periods of time as your baby sleeps and your body may feel like it's been hit by a truck.

In the hospital, you will fumble your way through your baby's first feedings, first diaper changes, and first bath. It is pretty emotional as you stare at that little face lying there next to you. But wait, I'm getting too emotional remembering those early days so I must switch gears and start talking about poo again. *"What the hell is that coming out of my baby's bum?"*

You read the books and they state that baby's first few bowel movements are called meconium, and you sort of drift through that not really knowing what that means or what to expect. *"It is black, oozing, sticky tar for crying out loud!!! That's what it is!"* Not anything you could possibly associate with any kind of regular bowel movement. And it does not wipe away easily. So bring some petroleum jelly with you and put some on your baby's bottom after each diaper change to make it easier to wipe the next time around. Let me be clear. I do not mean to put it on your baby's bum cheeks. Put the petroleum jelly right on the exit door.

Speaking of jelly, that's pretty much what your belly will feel like after giving birth. From a physical comfort perspective, I was ecstatic not to be pregnant anymore because I could breathe again. That abdominal pressure was gone so the soreness and labor discomfort were easily overlooked. My belly was immediately smaller but I still looked pregnant and would continue to look pregnant for some time. What was weird however was the feeling of my belly when I would walk. With every step, it would feel like Jell-o, swishing from side to side. *"No six-pack here baby, just a big swishy keg!"*

A minor point but it was important enough for me that I feel the need to include it here. I absolutely loved being served my meals in the hospital. Take full advantage of it. I know, you're probably thinking, *"Yuck, hospital food"*, but I enjoyed it all the same. Someone was taking care of me and all I had to do was sit back and eat. You will be so tired and busy for the next several months (or years) that it is so important to sit back and accept help from anyone if and when it is offered.

Other stuff you will discover in the first few days:

- Newborns are wobbly and they are hard to handle if you are a first-timer especially when you are trying to give them a bath. Be extra careful but don't worry, no one is judging you.

- Newborns may spit up what looks like frothy saliva. They are just clearing out their lungs. For both my babies, the nurses lifted their little beds up on one end, slightly elevating their head and also tilted their body slightly to one side.

- The stump left from the remains of the umbilical cord will get crusty and fall off in a few short days. Pat it dry after bathing your baby but no special attention is required.

- If this is your first child, you may be anxious about going home. If you have already gone through this before, you will be itching to get home. Different perspective, however regardless of what number child this is, the ride home from the hospital is always nerve-racking and probably the slowest, most conscientious driving you will ever experience.

Definitely some precious cargo on board so drive carefully.

CHAPTER 19

THEY JUST DON'T WORK!

I have so many feelings about breastfeeding. As the primary food source for the first months of my children's lives, I experienced all of these feelings at various points: Awkwardness, fear, insecurity, inadequacy, despair, discomfort, toe-curling pain, warmth, tenderness, love, sadness, and nostalgia. Let me explain a bit more.

With both children, within 30 minutes or so of giving birth, I was handed my child and encouraged to bring her to my breast to feed. There typically isn't any milk produced at this point but rather a yellowish substance called *colostrum* which is just what the baby needs. For my second child, this process was easy-peasy. I knew what to do and my breasts knew what to do. Babies automatically know what to do it seems. What an awkward feeling however the first time I did this. I was completely self-conscious, and I didn't have a freaking clue what I was doing. I could barely hold this tiny thing let alone feel comfortable in putting her to my breast. My heart was pounding in my chest. The nurse guided me on how to hold my breast, my baby moved in with her mouth open, she tried to latch on and then she popped right back off. We tried again. Nothing.

And so it went, every three hours or so, we would try again. Baby would get frustrated, cry, and then eventually go back to sleep. For days I couldn't tell if she was getting any nourishment but I did know that her weight was dropping. How did I know it was dropping? Because everything is tracked from the moment you give birth.

- How much does the baby weigh?

- How long is the baby?

- How big is the baby's head?

- What time did the baby eat? For how long? From which breast?

- Did the baby pee? How many times?

- Did the baby poo? How many times? What consistency? What color?

Just a quick aside on the capturing of data. The hospital provided me with a basic chart to track this while we were there and I tried to replicate these charts at home. Basic paper and pencil notes, check marks, you get the picture. I have however seen some amazingly elaborate charts from other parents and I am amazed at the dedication some people have to capture every possible statistic, input it into a spreadsheet, color-coded data, and graphs. I recall one proud father who wanted to share baby photos with a bunch of his friends so he forwarded an email with baby pictures which had been sent to him by his wife. Unfortunately for them, the email also had their baby's *Bowel Movement* spreadsheet attached. *"Wow! That's a lot of information."*

Anyway, back to my starving baby. We were in the hospital for two days and I was told that I was doing things properly but there was nothing coming out of my breasts. I thought this was supposed to be a natural, easy, organic process. With each passing day, I was growing more and more worried and my whole life revolved around figuring out how to keep my child from starving. *"God forbid I give her formula! Oh no, she will get confused and then never go back to breast milk."* I stressed in the hospital, then I stressed at home not knowing what to do, feeling that it was my fault and my breasts were just inadequate. They were failing my child.

An independent person by nature who knows how to fix things, so why couldn't I fix this? As you can probably tell, I am not the type of person who finds it easy to ask others for help. I felt like a failure but somehow got the courage to call a lactation specialist after a couple of days. It was the best decision I made. She was amazing and kind and she reassured me that everything was going to work out and told me that my milk hadn't come in yet. A light bulb went off in my head. *"Seriously? Isn't it just in there? Doesn't it start on its own? What's taking it so long?"* Apparently breast milk starts to flow as your baby suckles on the breast. Since my baby wasn't latching on there wasn't any kind of suckling happening therefore my body wasn't triggering this response. I had read that the suckling would increase my milk flow to satisfy my baby's growing needs however I always assumed that physiologically, my own body would automatically start the milk production. It doesn't. The solution in my case was to use a breast pump.

For the next three days, I would try to nurse my baby every 3-4 hours then I would give her one ounce of formula, put her back to bed and then use the breast pump to try and get things going. My physician recommended I supplement her feedings with formula because her weight had dropped by a couple of pounds and I trusted his judgement. From the time I gave birth, it took seven days for my body to begin producing milk. I had completely turned into myself, questioning everything, whether I should give up trying altogether, hating my useless breasts. All my angst was completely linked to the pressure of doing things perfectly for my child, whatever that really means. It was the longest, most depressing week of my life. Think about that though, it was just one week. That's a lot of pressure we put on ourselves.

In any case, they finally worked. There is however so much more to say about the breasts and what nursing does to them so let's begin.

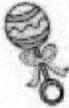

CHAPTER 20

BREASTFEEDING: THE BASICS

If you have chosen to breastfeed and everything is functioning properly (i.e. you are healthy and able to breastfeed, your baby is physically able to latch on) you will soon realize that what seems so unfamiliar at the beginning will become second nature fairly quickly although there may be some hiccups along the way. Here are some of the basics of breastfeeding.

POSITIONS

These can vary from the cradle hold, crossover hold, football hold, and side-lying hold.

- By far, when nursing my children, my go-to position was the *cradle hold*. This means that you hold your child sideways in your arms as if you are rocking them to sleep with your baby's head resting in the crook of your arm and their body facing slightly inwards towards you. If your baby's head is to the left, then the baby will feed from your left breast. Alternate sides with each feeding.

- In the first few weeks after birth, as my baby and I were trying to get the hang of breastfeeding, I used the *crossover hold* instead. This is fairly similar to the aforementioned cradle hold in the overall positioning of you and your baby with some slight modifications. With the crossover hold, you do not cradle your baby's head in the crook of your arm but rather use your opposite hand to support the baby's head and position it properly on your breast and the other hand is used to hold, direct and slightly compress your breast.

- For night-time feedings, or if I was tired during the day, I would lie down in bed on my side facing my baby, bring her close to my body, and she would nurse while lying down. Your baby nurses from the breast which is closest to the bed.

Night-time feedings can be so loving and peaceful as you sit with your baby quietly but they can also be long and tiring. Sometimes it can feel as if you are the only person awake in the entire neighborhood. Sitting in the glider in the nursery, I would get that tingly feeling in my body as I was slowly drifting off to la-la land and then suddenly I would jump in a panic. It scared me to think I could fall asleep, slump in the chair and smother my baby. That is why I much prefer the side-lying position. At least I was horizontal and could rest while feeding.

The first few months after giving birth, I had recurring nightmares of accidentally doing something that would hurt my child. I would have visions of slipping and falling down the stairs while holding my baby or of rolling onto my baby and smothering her as she slept next to me. It had me thinking at times that I might be losing my mind yet I was afraid to mention this to anyone. I jokingly asked another mom one day if she ever had these weird thoughts and to my relief she said yes. It made me feel so much better to know I wasn't alone. Hormones make you crazy!

• The final position, the *football hold*, is one I never used however is very useful for women who have had a C-section or a multiple birth. With this position, your baby is positioned to the side of your body, with their head facing your breast, your hand supporting their head up towards your breast, and their body tucked under your arm.

This position keeps the weight of your baby away from your abdomen which may be sore due to a C-section. If you are having twins and are concerned about how you will breastfeed two babies, the football hold allows you to feed both babies at the same time, with one baby on each breast.

ACCESSORIES

When breastfeeding, for all intents and purposes all you really need is your baby and your breasts. There are however a few things that can help the process.

- **Pillow**: If using the cradle position, your arms are what hold the baby. It will seem like you are feeding your baby all the time (at least every 2-3 hours and sometimes practically non-stop when they are going through a growth spurt) so your arms can get pretty tired and numb from being in the same position so frequently. You also want to sit as comfortable as possible so that your back does not start to ache. What can often happen is that your arms will get tired holding your baby up to your breast so you slowly begin to lower your arms closer to your lap and then dip your body forward bringing your breast closer to the baby. Bad idea. Bad for your back. It will already be sore from holding your baby all the time, don't exacerbate the problem. A nice thick standard pillow placed in your lap will help solve your problems. Your baby can rest on the pillow, and feed in a position which is comfortable for both of you.

- **Comfortable chair**: While I am not suggesting you drop a lot of money to get a new chair, it is important to have a comfortable spot to nurse your child. You can use a rocking chair, glider, bed or couch but I highly recommend having some sort of ottoman to rest your feet as well. Don't forget that you can also check out community garage sales, websites such as kijiji.com or your local classified ads for used baby gear.

  While many people don't necessarily choose a particular spot to breastfeed their baby, I do recommend having your own special place for feeding your baby. As your baby gets older and becomes more easily distracted by noises or older siblings you will appreciate having a calm, quiet, comfortable spot to go to.

- **Shawl**: There are a variety of products on the market to help mothers be more discreet when they are nursing in public (i.e. to hide their boobs from the horrified public who have obviously never seen a female breast before but I digress). These range from ponchos, to blankets, to slings. I discovered the most comfortable product to use just by accident when I was in a restaurant and didn't have a blanket with me. I instead used my *pashmina* scarf. It was long enough that I could drape it over the baby, my breast and my shoulder, loose enough that it provided me with viewing room to get my baby to latch on properly and soft enough that it wasn't hot or uncomfortable over the baby's head.

If you are going to spend some money, buy a few shawls in lively colors instead. You can still enjoy them even when your breastfeeding days are a thing of the past.

CLOTHING

Do you really need any special clothes when breastfeeding? No, not really, but here are some suggestions to make life a little bit easier.

- **Soft bras**: You will want a bra that is soft and comfortable against your breasts. Buy a few of them because things can get messy. You can opt for nursing bras with little hooks that open up to expose your nipples or a sports bra that can easily be slipped over or under your breast when feeding your baby.

- **Tank tops**: Tank tops became a fashion staple after having children. I still layer them with other shirts all the time. When I was breastfeeding, it was nice to be able to simply lower my tank top and bra and not have to expose my jelly belly to the world.

• **Zipper sweaters or button-down shirts**: When going out in public any such top just made things so much easier if I had to breastfeed because it would provide simple, discreet access to my boobs.

DIET

There is a lot of focus on what to eat when you are breastfeeding. Diet is a hot button topic regardless of whether or not you are a new mom. It is important to eat healthy meals, not just when breastfeeding but all the time. How do you define that however? For me it means to eat food that is real, you know, made out of real ingredients as opposed to food which is processed.

Be aware that your food choices will have an impact on your baby. Certain foods, including spicy foods or dairy products, may make your baby irritable (eg. change in poo consistency, more gas, more crying). Besides that, the only specific items you should avoid when breastfeeding are alcohol and excessive caffeine because they do find their way into your breast milk.

You will slowly start to lose your pregnancy weight once you have given birth and breastfeeding will help as it tightens your uterus and burns some extra calories. However, whenever I hear or read about some celebrity claiming their secret to losing baby weight is to breastfeed I want to scream. *"That's a load of crap!"* The secret to losing your baby weight is to eat good food, eat the right amount of calories and to exercise. Breastfeeding burns calories yes. Not enough to lose your pregnancy weight. Period.

Now go grab that little bundle of joy, have something to drink or a snack within reach, get yourself comfortable, and enjoy this amazing time with your baby. And don't forget to go to the washroom first because this could take awhile. There's nothing quite like the feeling of having to go (you know, really go, like number 2 go) and not wanting to interrupt your child's feeding. That's a perfect recipe for constipation and hemorrhoids. *"What? I never said that happened to me."*

CHAPTER 21

BREASTFEEDING: THE BAD STUFF

So my milk finally came in and before I knew it, my breasts were enormous. If you've never experienced this, it is quite shocking how engorged your breasts become. I'm talking adult-entertainment status. The downside however is that your breasts become swollen, hard, and uncomfortable. It can also be extremely painful.

The first few days after birth, as you and your baby are getting used to the process of breastfeeding, your baby may not always be latching on to your nipple properly. With an engorged breast, it makes it that much harder for the baby to latch on because your breast tissue is so hard and the nipple itself is so taut. This period of engorgement doesn't typically last too long, perhaps a few days; however there are certain things that you can do to ease some of the pain.

- Take a hot shower or apply heat to your breasts to soften your breast tissue and encourage letdown of your milk prior to feeding your child. I had a tube sock filled with rice that I would pop into the microwave for a couple of minutes to heat up and then I would lie down and place it on my breasts.

- Gently massage your breast and express some milk (either by hand or with a pump) prior to feeding in order to get your milk to start flowing. By the way, I never managed to express any milk by hand. Ever. Well, maybe just a dot.

- Place an ice pack (or something chilled) on your breasts after nursing to reduce some of the swelling.

- And most importantly, if you are committed to breast feeding, do not skip or shorten a feeding because your breasts will become more engorged and this can lead to infections such as mastitis. Never had this but many friends have and it is painful. Not to mention the antibiotics you will have to take.

If this is your first child, comparing notes with other moms can often be helpful but sometimes it can freak you out. Not all babies are the same in their feeding patterns and not all breasts are the same. Some babies will guzzle up milk in a few short minutes while others will suckle slowly for a really long time. For example, with my first child, feedings would often last 40 minutes to an hour. With my second child, 5 to 10 minutes maximum.

In addition to the discomfort of breast engorgement, there is also the issue of sore nipples. Just as I got the hang of breastfeeding and I thought it would be smooth sailing from then on, my nipples fell off. Honestly, what the hell was that all about? One minute, my nipples were slightly swollen and tender and the next minute I was experiencing toe-curling pain every time my baby would latch on. It was excruciating and everyone told me to apply a nipple cream to help ease the pain. The brand I used was *Lansinoh*. There are other brands but for the most part all of these products are lanolin-based. Every time I would apply the cream I would get so itchy that I wanted to rip off my nipples. I could not understand why this was happening. After a couple of weeks, the baby was better at latching on and my nipples had toughened up somewhat so I was in the clear from all the pain. I stopped using the cream and the itchiness went away. Well it turns out that lanolin is produced from the fleece of sheep and yours truly is allergic to wool. Do you see where I'm going with this? If, like me, you get itchy all over whenever you put on a wool sweater, you read it here, watch out for those nipple creams.

Finally there is the issue of leaking breasts. When we are pregnant, we go shopping trying to figure out what we will need for the baby, trying to decipher what is useful and what is just cute. With my first pregnancy, I stocked up on breast pads thinking them an absolute necessity and I never used them. I would hear other moms say how they had such an abundant flow of milk, how their milk would start flowing just hearing a baby cry out in public and I couldn't relate. I never had so much as a dot of wetness on my clothes. At around the 8-month mark however, as my baby started to sleep for longer stretches of time, my breasts would get engorged because she wasn't feeding as regularly. That's when I would often wake up to her early morning cries and be soaked through. So much for those breast pads. With my second child, it was a completely different story. The milk production was in high gear. My breasts were significantly less sore but what a mess!

CHAPTER 22

LET'S GO SHOPPING!

It can be so tempting and exciting to rush out and buy everything you see when you first find out you are expecting. There are however so many expenses that go along with having children and so many options of what to buy that you can often feel overwhelmed or just simply annoyed that you spent money on something that turned out to be absolutely useless. Please read on to see my thoughts on items which are worth every penny and others which are a complete waste of money.

TOP 10 ITEMS WORTH EVERY PENNY

1. **Stroller with Bucket Seat**: You will definitely need a stroller for any type of outing with the baby but keep in mind that you will also be putting this stroller in and out of your car frequently so you will want something that can fold easily. I highly recommend a stroller with a *one-hand* open/close mechanism because sometimes you will be stuck holding your

baby with the other hand. There are some strollers on the market that are absolutely beautiful in appearance but very difficult to manoeuvre when opening and closing. Try things out in the store before making your decision and don't be swayed solely on appearance. I had the *Quattro Tour Deluxe Travel System by Graco*. Definitely not the trendiest product on the market so you'll probably never glimpse a celebrity pushing one of these along but I have nothing negative to say about its performance. It was sturdy, easy to use, and way more economical.

2. **Baby monitor**: There are many options available and marketers do a great job of making the most expensive product seem like the best option by playing on a new parent's fears. With baby monitors you will find video options allowing you to see your baby from a distance. There are also motion sensing options allowing you to be alerted if your baby has stopped moving or breathing. This latter option will make you lose your mind and keep you in a constant state of panic. Don't even think about getting something like this. What you need is a baby monitor that is mobile so you can carry it with you anywhere and it must have a rechargeable base. Do not get anything with batteries because you will be constantly replacing them.

After so many years, I still use the monitor. It is a very handy tool to have around the house. For example, my husband and I will often be sitting outside with our friends in the summer after the children have gone to bed. With the monitor I can easily keep an *ear* on what's going on inside the house.

3. **Diaper Pail**: Unless you want your house to constantly smell like a bathroom disaster, you should invest in some sort of diaper pail. I had the *Diaper Champ by Baby Trend* which sealed really well so no odors escaped. It also used regular garbage bags so we didn't have to worry about purchasing specific garbage bags just for diapers.

4. **White-noise machine:** With my first child, whenever she struggled to fall asleep, I would blame it on our open-concept house for amplifying all noises. As I rocked her in my arms endlessly, I could hear my husband breathing downstairs. *"Why is he breathing so loud? Doesn't he know that I'm trying to get the baby to sleep? Does he really need to watch TV now? C'mon man, stop making so much noise!!!"* I was crazy ... I know.

With my second child however I discovered the white-noise machine. It was a clock-radio with different spa sounds like birds, rainfall, and ocean waves. With today's technology, there must certainly be an app which can achieve the same effect. The sounds were great for soothing my baby and for blocking out all the noises, even the sound of her older sister playing. An added bonus was that we could easily take it with us and it would help soothe her even when we were travelling.

5. **Baby carrier or sling:** A baby carrier is soothing to your child as well as great for reducing back strain for the person holding the child. I could do just about anything with my baby strapped on me. She was content to be with me and I wasn't breaking my back. It is funny how your body will adapt though. In the beginning, babies weigh practically nothing and yet holding them for long periods of time can be exhausting. Soon enough you will be lugging around a 25-pounder on your hip like it's nothing.

6. **Reclining high-chair:** Although it will be several months before you will need a high-chair to feed your baby, a reclining one can still be useful from very early on. If money or space is an issue, you will want to buy items that can do multiple-duty. A high-chair can serve as a seat for your baby. It needs to

recline however because your baby will not be able to sit properly for several months to come.

7. **Playard (also referred to as a playpen or Pack 'N Play®):** This serves so many purposes as your baby grows. Many playards come equipped with a bassinet so it can be the first place your baby sleeps when you bring them home. If you travel or visit family, you can easily bring it with you so that your baby has a place to sleep. Your baby can also play safely inside and it is always a great spot to plop baby down in when you have to do something and want to be certain that your baby cannot get out.

8. **Diaper shirts and front-closing sleepers:** Feel free to buy many of these as you will be using them all the time. For the first months at least, I do suggest you buy ones with the front closing snaps or zippers rather than the ones you button in the back or pull over the baby's head because they are just easier to manage. Babies are wobbly.

9. **Cool-mist humidifier:** You do not need anything extravagant but it is helpful to have a small, portable, cool-mist humidifier on hand. When your baby gets that first cold and is congested, it will break your heart to hear them struggling. The humidifier will make it easier for them to breathe.

10. **ExerSaucer®:** Babies do not need any special toys, especially not in the first few months, but an ExerSaucer® provides a fun, safe, stationary activity centre with attachments that babies can amuse themselves with while still taking in the action around them. Your baby can probably start using this at approximately 4 months although the detachable toys that come with it can be used even sooner to entertain your baby.

TOP 10 ITEMS THAT ARE A WASTE OF MONEY

If you have the money and think you need these items then go for it, but in my opinion, these are items you can very easily skip.

1. **Comforter and bumper pads**: Although these items are beautiful and there are so many different patterns and designs to choose from, they are simply not useful and are dangerous for your baby. Recommendations for safe sleeping habits for babies include putting them to sleep on their back. This has been shown to reduce the risk of SIDS (Sudden Infant Death Syndrome). *"How many times have I heard someone say, my mother put me to sleep on my stomach and look at me, I'm still alive? Ok great, so you weren't one of the sad stories but why would you want to risk that with your own child?"*

To further reduce any risk of suffocation, all soft, cushiony bedding materials should be removed from the baby's sleeping area. As for me, I received a beautiful set as a gift and it only ever came out of the closet when we were expecting company. *"What a waste of money!"*

2. **Bassinet**: Some people feel more comfortable putting their newborn to sleep close by in a bassinet. This is completely understandable. I did the same with my first child, using the bassinet in the playard, however I heard every single noise, sigh, gurgle that she made. Babies make a lot of noises when they sleep and this kept me up all night in a panic. After a couple of days, I moved her into the crib. Luckily I never spent the money on a separate bassinet.

3. **Toys:** Don't waste your money on anything too fancy, sophisticated or anything claiming to enhance your child's brain activity. Particularly in the first six months or so because they really are not able to do too much. Snuggle with your baby, dangle items over their head and watch them try to grab or kick their legs. They will most probably want to put everything in their mouths so watch out for small items. The plastic bulb on the turkey baster as well as a plastic medicine dropper (*"It was clean, don't*

worry!") kept both my children occupied for long periods of time.

Once they are more mobile, a cupboard or drawer of Tupperware and wooden spoons will come in handy.

4. **Bottle sterilization kit:** Just grab a pot, boil some water, and place whatever needs sterilization (bottles, pacifiers, breast pump) in the boiling water for a few minutes.

5. **Fancy clothes:** There are so many beautiful articles of clothing available that it can be hard not to scoop up everything in sight. The reality is that newborn babies grow so quickly and many outfits will never be worn even if you do make a concerted effort to dress them up regularly. Whenever I see babies that are all decked out in fancy outfits, they seem very uncomfortable, particularly in the first few months. Cotton and comfortable is the way to go.

6. **Shoes:** Your baby's feet will not even fit properly into shoes for many months to come so even though they are cute, you should realize that most children shoes are as expensive as adult shoes, can be easily lost as you are pushing your baby along in the stroller and they serve no functional purpose whatsoever.

7. **Breastfeeding pillow:** These pillows are available at many different price points but as I mentioned previously, a good old regular pillow will do the job just as well, if not better. And with a regular pillow, you can easily slip off the pillowcase and toss it in the wash.

8. **Wipe warmer:** If you have chosen to use cloths, this may not be relevant however if you will be using disposable wipes (*"Yes, they are convenient"*), buying a separate device to keep these wipes warm is somewhat extravagant. I suppose that some babies are perhaps more sensitive to temperature than others but I think this gadget was invented to make parents feel all warm and fuzzy that they are taking good care of their baby. Save the money on the warmer and buy more wipes.

9. **Bottle warmer:** These gadgets take forever to warm up the milk. Pop that bottle in the microwave, give the milk a good shake to ensure there are no hot spots, feed baby and get him or her back to sleep. The person with the bottle warmer is still waiting for their milk to heat up.

10. **Expensive breast pump:** Depending on how long you will be staying home with your baby, you may need to use a breast pump to store milk for your

baby for when you are at work perhaps. If this is the case then you should get a fairly robust electric breast pump but prices can range from several hundred dollars to upwards of a thousand. That is a big investment to make so I would recommend you do your research and see whether you can rent a hospital-grade breast pump in your area. This typically involves buying the accessories for a nominal amount (i.e. anything that comes into contact with you and your milk) and then you rent the machine itself for a couple of dollars a day.

For everyone else, who just want to supplement breastfeeding with the occasional bottle, a simple breast pump should do the job fairly well. Why spend hundreds of dollars? Remember, you are feeding a baby not an entire sports team. Some new moms can get a little bit excessive on how much breast milk they store. I have looked into some freezers and have been left speechless by the number of little bags of milk that were in there.

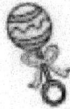

CHAPTER 23

BABY OLYMPICS

From the moment your baby is born, everything will be measured. Your newborn's length, weight, and head circumference will be recorded and he or she will be assigned an Apgar score. This score reflects your baby's overall condition in the following categories: Appearance (color), Pulse (heartbeat), Grimace (response to stimulation), Activity (muscle tone), and Respiration (breathing). At all subsequent doctor appointments, your baby's measurements will be tracked and they will be assigned a percentile ranking for length, weight, and head circumference. If your baby is in the 70th percentile for weight, for example, then you will know that, on average, your baby weighs more than 70% of all same-sex babies of the same age at that time.

I can still easily recall both my daughters' exact birth weight, but all these other measurements have been cleansed from my memory. What is funny however is that at the time, when my baby was being continuously measured at every doctor's appointment, I was amazed at how so many other parents, who were in the same boat as us, were obsessed with these numbers. I would be asked repeatedly what percentile they were in. No big deal, right? But both my daughters were long and fairly heavy, particularly my oldest daughter, who is often the tallest person in her class, and they were regularly in the 100+ percentile. Some parents, whose children were smaller, would seemingly apologize for their child's ranking. As if they somehow failed a test. Frivolous stuff but I'm always amazed at people's need to compare and compete.

A good friend of mine, who always makes me laugh with her stories, told me that her sister-in-law, who had a child at the same time as her, was obsessed with keeping track of both their babies' measurements, continuously striving for her baby to *win*. When my friend stopped sharing the information with her, she tried to get the information directly from their doctor (both babies had the same paediatrician). Sounds wacky to me and we can blame it on the hormones. However, maybe it's not the hormones; maybe it's the ever- present strive for perfection in our society.

CHAPTER 24

ROCK-A-BYE BABY

Here are the facts: Your baby may be the child who naps regularly, doesn't require much assistance to get to sleep nor to stay asleep, and who sleeps through the night after only just a few weeks. Some babies are truly fantastic sleepers. But you also need to know that your child may be the child who wants to be rocked endlessly, wakes up from his or her nap after only a few short minutes, reacts to every sound, and does not sleep through the night at 2 months, 6 months or even after a year. Some children continue to wake you at night for years to come. This is definitely possible and it is not uncommon. I have experienced both extremes and I can definitely say that a sleeping baby makes for a happy mommy. When your baby sleeps easily and for long stretches of time at night, this reduces so much tension, anxiety and fatigue in parents and makes for a much happier baby as well.

There are so many books and websites focused on how to ensure your baby develops good sleeping habits and while there are some interesting ideas and suggestions, I honestly believe that what works for one child will not necessarily work for another. In addition, I also truly believe that sometimes nothing works. I have *("had?")* a lot of patience for my children and I was ready to endure crying over multiple nights, not to run and pick them up immediately, to maintain a good routine, to observe my child for signs of sleepiness so that I could put her to bed before she got overtired. *"Wait! How many yawns was that?"* For one of my daughters at least, sleep was never something that we mastered. I was definitely not a baby whisperer. Just remembering this time makes me anxious. Here are some sleeping experiences that many parents can relate to.

- I would be nursing my first born, Eva, and her eyes would slowly close, she would drift off to sleep. *"Now what? Do I wake her? Do I burp her? She's supposed to learn to put herself to sleep rather than fall asleep nursing, isn't she?"* After much trial and error, my husband and I concluded that this child was not going to fall asleep on her own in her crib. All the experts are cringing but it is what it is. Let me describe what would happen next.

I would walk to the side of the crib with her sound asleep in my arms, gently lower her towards the mattress and, you guessed it, she would start screaming bloody murder. My heart would sink but I would try again. I would hold her closely, maybe rock her gently in my arms, sing lullabies over and over and over *"Close your eyes. Go to sleep. I will see you in the morning. Close your eyes. Close your eyes. Close your f@%*ing eyes!"* and finally she would be asleep again. I would walk to the side of the crib, gently lower her onto the mattress and, if she didn't start screaming, I would take a deep breath and with painstaking precision, remove both my hands from her body as gently as possible. *"Ok, so far so good"*. Retreating from her room in slow motion trying not to make a sound, I would typically make it to the bedroom door with her still sleeping soundly. The moment I smelled victory and turned my body to walk away, she would start screaming again. *"Shit!"* This would go on multiple times every single day nearly sending me over the edge.

• When Eva was about three months old, I discovered the magic of Michael Bublé. I had seen him interviewed on television discussing his latest album, *It's Time,* and I fell in love with that voice. I bought the CD that same day and in the evening, after dinner, we put it on for the first time and discovered its magical powers. From the first few notes of *Feeling Good*, my baby would be in a trance. By *Quando, Quando, Quando*, she was in a deep sleep. We listened to Michael Bublé so much that I will forever associate his music with my oldest daughter.

Our youngest, Gia, was a much better sleeper. Her signals were easier to read. She too liked the occasional lullaby but she preferred to be put in bed while still awake. She would gurgle, stare at the mobile, and drift off to sleep all by herself. She did however also have a sleep CD but it was reserved for car rides. The sweet gentle voice of Jack Johnson on *Sleep through the Static* worked wonders on her.

- While I was living through the sleep craziness with my firstborn, my brother and sister-in-law were also having some wild sleeping adventures with their own brand new baby. I remember visiting them with my colicky baby and observing their child who never cried. "*Seriously! Does this kid ever cry?*"

Alas, they didn't have it easy in the sleep department either. He started off tiny but within a couple of months, he was a fairly large baby and hated being cradled. My brother or his wife would hold their baby up vertically and slow danced with him for practically the entire Elton John Greatest Hits trying to get him to sleep. Just remembering this cracks me up of course because I didn't have to endure it. *"Hold me closer tiny dancer..."* I'm sure they have burned that CD by now.

- As Eva grew a few months older she developed the habit of rubbing her earlobe to fall asleep. I should mention that this was in addition to all the other sleep crutches (rocking, singing, music, etc.) This is pretty common it seems, almost like using a pacifier I guess, but eventually she expanded her horizons and any earlobe would do. Neither one of her grandmothers was ever able to get her to fall asleep until Eva discovered their earlobes. Sometimes, at family gatherings, we all reminisce how we were handcuffed to this sweet baby by the grasp she had on our earlobes.

- Being our firstborn, it was very easy to keep the house quiet when Eva was asleep. This wasn't necessarily intentional, it just happened. We didn't have another child to make noise and we didn't have a lot of people coming and going from our house since both our families and most of our friends at that time lived out of town. So whenever we had company or when we travelled to visit others, sleep time was stress time. And I should mention that it's one thing to be stressed in your own environment with no witnesses but a whole other ball game when you are around others who are looking at your crying baby, who won't fall asleep, and your insecurities are constantly forcing you to come up with some ridiculous excuse as to why your baby keeps waking up every 20 minutes crying.

I remember holding her, trying to comfort her but so worried that we were disturbing others that I would sit in the bathroom with the fan switched on or rock her near the stovetop hood fan, practically shoving her up into it, to try and soothe her with the humming sounds. Sometimes this worked and sometimes we just got the comments from others "Just let her cry, she'll learn!" I tried it, for several days, heard a lot of endless crying, and I didn't like it.

- Stroller rides, the perfect sleep solution for many difficult sleepers, didn't work for my children. I walked and walked but sleep never came except for that one time, which we so clearly remember, where we were walking towards the beach in Cape Cod, there was a wonderful ocean breeze, Eva was sitting in a stroller and was about 8 months old. The grownups were chatting up a storm, enjoying the weather, the view, the fact that the children were quiet when I noticed that Eva was leaning sideways, fast asleep. In an umbrella stroller of all things.

I hope I haven't scared you but all of this is exhausting to think about. You need to be strong. You can handle anything that comes your way because it will pass or at least become tolerable. If your baby is a good sleeper, count your blessings.

To my sweet girl, you made us work hard but I loved you and will always love you so deeply even though you brought me to the brink of sanity. Perhaps you even pushed me over a little bit.

CHAPTER 25

JUST MAKE HER STOP!

Before you have children, you may hear people talking about their colicky baby and act like you sort of know what they are talking about but really you don't know and quite frankly, you don't really care. And then one day, you have a baby and you think that you have a good little routine going and then the baby starts to cry and you try to figure out what your baby needs. *"Is baby hungry? Does baby have a dirty diaper? Is baby hot? Is baby sleepy? Does baby have gas? No, no, no, no and no. Now what?"* You try rocking your baby, you try singing to your baby, you take your baby for a stroll, but hour after hour your baby continues to cry and fuss until you think your head is going to explode. That is the definition of colic. I swear. Look it up.

I was blessed with two colicky babies who would start to cry at around 5 or 6 o'clock in the evening every day. This wasn't regular crying which I felt relatively in control of. Instead it was crying that made me feel helpless because it would go on for about four hours every night. With both children, colic started at around the six week mark and I remember this because I was travelling alone with my first daughter at the time and I was freaking out not knowing what was happening. With both, it lasted for about three months. I do not claim that any of the following makes sense but here are some of the things that we did to help us cope through this trying time.

1. Strap baby into the baby carrier and keep them close to you. Vacuuming at the same time seemed to help as well. The noise of the vacuum cleaner would calm their cries and often put them to sleep. Perhaps this is not so good for their ears but at the time, you do what you have to do.

2. I would put baby in the bucket seat and just swing her gently back and forth. This got tiring very quickly. My husband used to take over often and he added his little twist of walking up and down the stairs with the baby. Repeatedly. He was convinced that the baby liked this. I thought he was nuts.

3. In extreme cases, I would put the baby in the car and go for a ride. Once she was asleep, I would pop the bucket seat out the car and bring her into the house.

And in case you were wondering, I wouldn't take her out of the bucket seat. I worried so much about this. I Googled it. Was I doing any damage to her by leaving her in the seat? After several failed attempts at transferring her to her crib however, I decided that that was where she would stay until she woke up. Maybe she got a little cramped in that position but referring back to point #1, you do what you have to do.

4. I occasionally resorted to using the baby swing at top speed. The slower speed just annoyed them but top speed probably freaked them out a little bit so that they quieted down for a while.

5. When I felt absolutely helpless after hours of listening to crying, I would pass the baby over to my husband and head into the bathroom, turn on the fan, climb into the tub, run a bath and stick my head under the water for a little while. The sound of the running water was the only way to block out the crying sounds. I would always know when my husband was reaching his breaking point because he would hover outside the bathroom door with our crying baby until I heard. Sometimes you just have to put your baby down, walk away and let them cry for awhile or else you are going to lose it.

6. The ultimate go-to strategy for soothing our youngest was a recommendation from a co-worker. He said to hold our crying baby and sit on an exercise ball. This would relieve any strain from constantly holding our child and the rocking motion from the ball would stop her cries. I was sceptical at first but it really helped. I was still trapped holding a baby for long periods of time but at least the crying had stopped. After a few days, we modified this technique by popping our baby into the bucket seat and then bouncing her on top of the exercise ball. This way, she would fall asleep and we could then gently place her on the floor and let her sleep for awhile.

Perhaps everyone is judging me for doing these things but for a few months it seemed that my sole objective was to win the war on crying. It was hard and I don't know who won that battle but before you know it, it was over, gone ... but not forgotten.

CHAPTER 26

THE BASICS ... AND THEN SOME!

The routine: From the moment you give birth, your life will become regimented. As previously mentioned, some people can be extreme in how closely they monitor every feeding, every nap or every bowel movement, but even if you are relatively carefree, there are certain things that need to happen every few hours or so whether you like it or not. This includes feeding and burping your baby, changing his or her diaper, entertaining them for a bit (which can include activities as simple as snuggling, massaging, stretching or just making silly faces) and then putting them down to sleep again. This cycle repeats itself multiple times a day in the first few months with the *awake* time gradually increasing as your baby gets older.

While this is not etched in stone, as a general guideline you can expect that in the first weeks, each cycle will go somewhat as follows:

- Baby will wake up.

- You will feed baby. Bottle feeding will typically be quicker but breastfeeding could take anywhere from 10 minutes up to an hour. Often your baby will fall asleep as the feeding is ending.

- You will burp baby. Even if your baby falls asleep during feeding, you really should burp them not only from a health perspective but really to save yourself the headache when they wake up in a few minutes crying because they are uncomfortable in their tummy.

- You will change baby's diaper.

- You will play with baby for a few minutes.

- Baby will go back to sleep. Since babies get hungry every two to three hours, depending on how quick the previous steps were completed, your baby may nap for one to two hours. Or in my case, 20 minutes.

As your baby gets older, they will typically settle into a routine where they nap once in the morning and once in the afternoon. With all this sleeping, do not be surprised when the back of your baby's head starts to develop a little bald spot from repeatedly resting in the same position. Some babies even develop what is referred to as cradle cap. This is a condition common in young infants where they develop scaly, flaky patches on their scalps. A little olive oil on the head prior to shampooing seems to help.

Bathing: Bathing a newborn can be somewhat tricky. A newborn is just a floppy little person that can't do much with their body just yet and introducing soap and water makes things quite slippery. The routine that I found worked for us was to use a baby bathtub suctioned right onto our bathroom counter. I could have put it right in the bathtub but then I would have had a sore back from leaning over the edge of the tub. I would wet a washcloth and wash baby's eyes and mouth first with some warm water, put a little bit of baby body wash on a washcloth and gently rub it in her hair first and then over her body. I used a cup which I would fill with water from the sink and pour it over her to rinse away the soap from her hair and the front of her body. Then I used my left hand to rest her body forward on my hand while I rinsed her back.

Once my daughters were able to get in a sitting position, probably at around four months, I switched them to a bath ring. This is a brilliant invention and very inexpensive. You put this in the bathtub and bathe your baby right in there without fear of them slipping. We had plenty of laughs bathing our daughters and watching them playing with their toys and the soap bubbles.

Medical Stuff:

- If you will be breastfeeding, your baby may require **Vitamin D** drops depending on where you live and how much exposure to the sun your baby will have. Speak with your physician to see whether this is necessary. My babies loved the Vitamin D. They would suck it back like nobody's business.

- **Immunization**: Over the next several months and years, your doctor will recommend an immunization schedule for your child against several diseases including but not limited to measles, mumps, rubella, chicken pox, hepatitis. There is so much you can read about this subject with a large community of people completely opposed to vaccinations. While I do not want to necessarily enter this debate, I will say that both my children have received the full immunization regimen. I am not a doctor but I do have a graduate degree in science. My point is that some of the arguments against vaccination are completely ludicrous and not based on any scientific fact. *"Confirmation bias anyone?"* As with most things, there is some risk, but in my opinion the benefits of protecting my child from these diseases far outweighs the risk of possible immunization side effects.

- **Baby acne**: Do not be surprised if your baby develops a bad case of acne within a few weeks of birth. While doctors say that not all babies develop acne, obviously both my daughters did and I have the pictures to prove it. *"So much for baby smooth skin."* With my firstborn, I remember noticing a little tiny mark on her face and then, in what seemed like only a few hours, her face was entirely covered with little red and white pimples. This clears up all by itself in a few weeks and doesn't require any special care or products.

- **Roseola**: While babies are susceptible to viruses, just as we all are, roseola is defined by 3 to 4 days of high fever and irritability. With both my children, this was their first fever and it can be quite scary. While many parents may not remember the term roseola, most will remember the time their baby had a fever and then suddenly developed a rash all over, particularly on their *trunk* as my doctor would say referring to the upper body, neck, and upper arms. That's what I remember ... spots everywhere.

- **Swollen breasts in newborns**: With all the estrogen hormones transferred from mother to baby during pregnancy and childbirth, it is possible for newborns, both female and male, to have swollen breasts. This is perfectly normal and subsides over the next few weeks to a year as the estrogen levels absorbed from the mother deplete and your baby's own hormone system begins to mature.

- **Vaginal bleeding in newborns**: Following similar reasoning, it is possible that a newborn girl may experience vaginal bleeding in the first weeks after birth.

I had absolutely never heard of this and was absolutely unprepared when, one day, as I was changing my newborn daughter's diaper, I saw blood. As you can imagine, I freaked out and my heart started racing with fear. A quick Google search today produces many hits on this subject and would quickly appease a worried parent. On that night however, over eight years ago, the internet took quite some time to give me the answers I was looking for.

Three years later, when the same thing happened with our second daughter, it was my husband who was changing her diaper. Obviously his power of recollection is not quite as strong as mine *("or any normal human being for that matter")* because he started screaming for me to come upstairs. When I reacted calmly to what he was showing me and told him it was no big deal, he was shocked and honestly couldn't remember the anguish we had felt only a few short years before. *"How could he not remember? I just don't get it."*

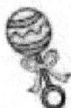

CHAPTER 27

LET'S GET BUSY

What could I possibly say about sex? Things can get tricky at times but isn't everything related to sex complicated at some point or another? Communication is always important in any relationship but the added burden of trying to get pregnant, being pregnant, or having a newborn, mixed in with a healthy dose of hormones, can make this a difficult path to navigate. Let's break it down.

Pre-Conception

In order to get pregnant the old-fashioned way, sexual intercourse will be required. This is fun. For most. Assuming you had a healthy sex life before, trying to get pregnant shouldn't change things. But sometimes it does. Stress, performance anxiety, fear, any number of factors could start creeping into you or your partner's sub conscience and this could zap some of the fun out of it.

If you don't get pregnant within a few months of trying, all your thoughts can become consumed with sex. How often should we do it? When should we do it? What position? Is there something wrong?

During Pregnancy

Once you are pregnant, your sex life could go back to normal or you may suddenly find that you or your partner start feeling uncomfortable about having sex.

From a woman's perspective, there are physiological and psychological changes taking place which may help or hinder her sexual urges.

- Morning sickness may hinder bedroom action. *"Nothing like nausea to get me in the mood."*

- Fatigue may also hinder bedroom action or it may reduce your inhibitions as you let your partner have his way with you while you rest.

- Your body is changing day by day and you may feel less attractive with these changes. On the other hand, you may feel sexier with more curves and larger breasts.

- Surging hormones may have you fantasizing about sex all the time or drain you of all desire with your focus solely on the baby inside you.

Your partner will also be going through a roller coaster of emotions and there is no way to know how that will affect the libido. For some, the pregnant female body is a turn-on and it can feel like he is sleeping with another person without actually cheating on you. The extra curves are something new to discover and your partner may have a hard time keeping his hands off of you.

There is the opposite extreme of course. Some men are completely not attracted to the pregnant female body which can cause problems in a relationship if their partners are made to feel guilty for being pregnant.

There are also those who feel uncomfortable with the idea that there is a baby in there. The funniest sub-category of these men are the ones who are afraid that they will damage or hit their baby's head during sex. *"Seriously, how big do you think you are?"*

Post-Partum
Six weeks. That number again. Physicians typically recommend women wait six weeks post-partum before engaging in sexual intercourse in order to promote healing and reduce the risk of infection. And it seems that many men are highly aware of this six week milestone.

Just as every pregnancy, labor, and delivery is different, so is the feeling of desire that women may or may not experience in the weeks after giving birth. For some women, everything gets back to normal fairly quickly while for others it takes some time.

Fear of pain *down there* may obviously dampen your mood. Your lady parts are a bit mangled, it's true, however many other factors, which may or may not have been anticipated, can also come into play. For example:

- Waking up at random hours throughout the night can drain you of the energy required to get your brain and body revved up for sex.

- Your breasts may also be sore and the thought of sexual contact can be frightening.

- Your breasts are also perhaps your baby's food source and thinking of them engaging in sexual acts can be weird. I felt as if I was cheating on my baby. And that was just the emotional aspect. *"What the hell happens if they leak?"*

- Hormonal changes can affect your mood making you happy one minute and teary the next. They can also reduce natural secretions making intercourse somewhat uncomfortable.

- Feeling pressure from your partner to perform can most definitely be a turn off. *"Back off and go change a diaper!"*

- Sometimes you just don't want to be touched. You spend your day with a newborn attached to your body and you may just want to reclaim some of your own space.

- Knowing that there is a baby in the house, perhaps sleeping right there next to you, can be a buzz kill and it may take some time to adjust to the idea that you no longer have the place all to yourselves. For years to come, your lovemaking will most certainly take place with others in the house but hopefully unaware of what is going on. *"Did my parents have sex while I was sleeping in the next room? Gross!"*

- Physical changes down there can also have a positive impact. With things, let's say, slightly stretched, there may be less friction or discomfort and with increased blood flow, even more sensitivity to pleasure.

As with all the changes you encounter throughout this entire process, communication is the key to preventing things from getting out of hand. If you don't feel like getting busy with your partner then you need to say so. A loving partner will most certainly understand. You are a mommy now, with new emotions, more aware of your own body, less inhibitions, more woman. In due time, with a little bit of planning and effort, sex after babies can be better than it ever was before.

CHAPTER 28

I'M SHEDDING LIKE A DOG

With all the physical changes that your body goes through during pregnancy, childbirth and post-partum, who really expects to be dealing with hair loss as well? I never knew this was something women may experience after giving birth until I visited a childhood friend a few months after she had given birth. The back of her sweater was a disaster. Long dark hairs were everywhere and I found myself constantly picking at her to clean the hairs away. She told me that her hair had just started falling out and she didn't know why. Well luckily nothing was wrong. At least from a health perspective that is. The shower drain however was a whole other problem.

During pregnancy, some women may suddenly find that they have super thick hair, more than usual, and this is because high levels of estrogen in the body prolong the growing phase of hair. In other words, more hair is growing than is falling or in the resting phase. For me this meant "commercial hair" if I bothered to fix it but most of the time, it was just tied up in a ponytail. About six months after birth however, as the hormone levels began to adjust, all this extra hair started to fall out. Things got pretty messy for awhile. This wasn't your typical kind of hair loss where a few hairs come out in your brush. The hair was everywhere. It was coming out in clumps in my brush, all over my cream-colored bathroom tiles, in my shower drain, on my pillow, everywhere. *"Where's the Drāno?"*

CHAPTER 29

I CHANGED MY MIND

Now that those early years, *survival-mode years* as I like to call them, are behind me, I feel nostalgic when I think of my girls as babies. But if I close my eyes and remember what the first year with a newborn was like, I clearly recall the occasional time or two (or three) where I thought to myself *"I changed my mind. I just can't do this anymore. Can we bring her back?"*

With babies comes unconditional love but there also comes a ton of work, routine physical labor that some days, many days, made me feel like I was going off the deep end. I have never felt more exhausted in my entire life than I did in the first year after my first child. Hopefully you will have more people around for support because you are signing up for some heavy hitting. This is the exhausting, repetitive, never-ending routine stuff I remember from the first year. Don't worry,

I wasn't miserable all the time. I just want you to be aware so that you can feel free to bitch and moan about it from time to time and not feel like you are the only mom who isn't always in a Mary Poppins cheery mood.

- Constant diaper changes. Lay baby down, open diaper flaps, wipe the mess, apply any cream if necessary, roll up diaper, toss, pull out fresh diaper, open diaper, place it under baby's bum, position diaper, pull flap over front, attach sides. Over and over. Using a low estimate of three diaper changes per day, each day, for two and half years (and probably more), you will be changing over 2,700 diapers.

- Breastfeeding. Every three hours at a minimum but usually more like every two hours.

- Endless feedings. Buy the food, prepare the food, sit baby in chair, bring food to baby's mouth, trick baby into opening their mouth, pick food up off the floor, pick up food or bowls that baby keeps throwing on the floor, washing bibs, wiping down the high chair, wiping floor after feeding, washing all the plastic spoons, bowls, cups, bottles, pacifiers. My fingertips were so dry from all the washing.

Many parents are in such a rush to start feeding their baby solids and I am pretty sure this is because it's something new to do but be forewarned, it is much more labor intensive.

- Crying. This wears you out but amazingly you will probably develop a higher level of tolerance with any future babies.

- Putting baby to sleep, multiple naps throughout the day then again at night time, then maybe a few times in the middle of the night.

- Soothing, rocking, singing, tippy toeing out of the room.

- Baby talk.

- Endless walks with the stroller.

- Frequent washing of clothes from the messy feedings, spit up or the lovely explosive bowel movements that shoot up all over the baby's back.

- Bath time. Every single day. *"Please! Can't we just skip a day of bath time?"*

- Constantly lifting baby in and out of the crib, bath, car seat or stroller. My lower back still hasn't recovered.

Somehow though, we manage to do this every day, for many days and years, caring for these little monsters we created. Some days were amazing, some days were torture but I wouldn't trade them for anything. I'll leave it for my memories though because I wouldn't want go back. When I had a baby and I felt overwhelmed, there was always someone who would tell me "You think things are hard now, just wait until your child is older. Things are 100 times harder." Well, they were wrong. The first year was the hardest, both physically and emotionally. I need to go rest now; I'm tired just remembering it all.

CHAPTER 30

TIME FOR DINNER

After the first couple of months, you and your baby will probably be experts at feedings. Reading their signals will become second nature and if not, you will probably try to pop your breast (or the bottle) in their mouth when they cry and your baby will very quickly let you know if that is what they were looking for by either ravenously guzzling down the milk, or by pushing that nipple back out and showing no interest.

Eventually, babies are physically ready to eat solid foods. After 4 or 5 months approximately, they are able to sit up in a chair, they produce more saliva which helps with digestion, they are able to swallow and use their tongue to transfer food into their mouth and they are able to turn their head to indicate that they are full. In addition to being physically ready to eat, babies also require additional nutritional content besides what is available through breast milk or formula (eg. Iron, vitamin C). This is why, by month 6 or 7, it is important to begin feeding your baby solid foods in order for them to continue developing in a healthy manner.

When exactly you should introduce solid foods into your baby's diet is not written in stone and even if you have set a specific milestone as to when you plan on introducing solids, you may need to adjust based on your baby's development. In my opinion however, more often than not, that date changes because you desperately want to change up the daily routine a little bit and you have convinced yourself that your baby is *starving* when you see them licking their lips or staring at food when grownups are eating. Don't rush however because while it is fun to see baby's reaction to eating something new, starting too early may just be a waste of food, it can limit your milk supply, it will not make your baby sleep through the night (sorry), it is more expensive, and overall, it is much more work. Even if you choose to purchase pre-made commercial baby food, there is still a lot of mess and the corresponding clean up associated with feedings. As well as the horrific change to their bowel movements. Breastfed baby poo has nothing on solid food baby poo. *"Could somebody please open a window?"*

CHAPTER 31

FEEDING MADE EASY

It is finally time to give your baby something besides milk. How exciting! It really is. You just can't wait to see your baby open that adorable little mouth expectantly as you bring that cute little spoon towards them. I'll let you in on a secret though. It isn't always so easy to get them to open that little mouth of theirs. Sometimes you won't be able to scoop up the food fast enough for your baby but other times, you will find yourself resorting to making funny faces, funny noises, tricking them, just about anything to get them to open wide. It's fun either way but don't make yourself crazy with what to feed your baby.

There are so many books and blogs promising hundreds of quick, easy, and nutritious recipes for your baby. *"Hundreds! Who needs that many recipes? Are we opening a restaurant for babies?"* On the other hand, many people choose to feed their baby commercially prepared baby food. There are rows and rows of jars at your local grocery store filled with fruits, vegetables and various meat combinations readily available. As I've mentioned before, when it comes to diet, I am not a big proponent of any type of pre-packaged food. Then again I do enjoy cooking but I don't think preparing baby food requires any advanced culinary skills. Here are my suggestions for making healthy foods that do not require a lot of money, effort or creativity.

IN THE BEGINNING (6 - 7 months)

- It is recommended that you introduce one food (a single ingredient) at a time to your baby's diet to ensure your baby has no allergic reaction (eg. rash, swelling, runny nose, difficulty breathing, gas, diarrhea). Wait about 3-4 days before introducing another food.

- **Iron-fortified baby cereals**: There are many commercial cereal brands available but my brand of choice was *Milupa*. I loved all the flavours. It is typically recommended that you begin with a single ingredient cereal with rice being the most common first choice. Other options include oatmeal, barley and wheat cereals. The cereal is mixed with either water or breast milk, should be more liquid than solid and only 1-2 teaspoons of dry cereal are all that is needed in the first few days.

- You can start to introduce **fruits and vegetables** as well. There are so many options to choose from allowing you to introduce your baby to a variety of flavours, from sweet to savoury, expanding their pallet and hopefully avoiding a picky eater as they grow older.

- Fruit options include: apple, pear, banana, mango, peaches, plums, and apricots. These are simple to prepare. Depending on how ripe the fruit was, I would sometimes boil the fruit for a couple of minutes to soften then I would purée, and freeze into portions using ice cube trays. If you choose not to freeze, the freshly prepared food should be refrigerated and will last for 3-4 days. Freezing the prepared food however, allows you to mix things up when it's feeding time without worrying that food will spoil or go to waste. Pop the frozen portions into freezer bags and you will have a variety of foods to choose from at your disposal with each portion corresponding to roughly 1 tablespoon of food.

As your baby gets older, you can introduce fruits with seeds such as kiwi and berries while also gradually making the food lumpier. By about nine months, your baby will be able to chew soft foods or finely chopped foods even with no teeth. Their gums are strong.

- Vegetable options include: carrots, peas, squash, sweet potato, zucchini, beans, asparagus and broccoli which I would also boil, purée, and freeze.

MEAT AND ALTERNATIVES (8 months)

- Once you have introduced your baby to a variety of cereals, fruit and vegetables, you can offer iron-rich foods including meat, poultry, fish, egg yolks, and legumes.

- Meat options include chicken, beef, veal, lamb, and pork. These foods are prepared in a similar manner to the fruits and vegetables but it takes longer since the meat must cook through. Fancy preparations are neither necessary nor required. Simply place a portion of meat in boiling water, cook through, purée and freeze. No need for any seasoning or oils.

- Alternatives to meat include egg yolks (egg whites should not be introduced until your baby is a year old), beans and lentils. For eggs, boil in water until they are hard cooked, remove the egg white, and mash up the yolk. Depending on your baby's eating development, you can choose to mix the yolk slightly with breast milk or water to make it runnier or simply chop it up into small pieces. Beans or legumes should be boiled until tender, then puréed.

As your baby's diet expands to include a variety of new foods, you will notice a change to their bowel movements. Different foods do different things to their digestive systems and impact some babies more than others. At a high level, you can assume the following:

- Diapers will smell more.

- The consistency of your baby's poo will change. Less *mushy*, more like the real stuff.

- Bananas, Rice, Apples and Toast (B.R.A.T.) can constipate which will be helpful to remember if your baby has diarrhea. On the other hand, you may find yourself in the same situation I did a day after my baby ate a lot of bananas. I noticed her forcing to go to the bathroom and she suddenly started screaming bloody murder. I didn't know what was wrong but I took off her diaper and saw her poo stuck in her bum. She was all swollen and in so much pain. This wasn't mushy baby poo. It was, you know, grown up stuff. *"Oh my goodness! What am I supposed to do?"* I quickly put some Vaseline around her bum, grabbed some wipes and gently pushed down around her swollen skin to help slowly release her poop. *"That's right everybody. I used my hands to physically pull out a piece of crap from my baby's bum. Crisis averted. Lovely".*

FINGER FOODS (9 – 12 months)

At about 9 months, your baby will probably start showing an interest in grabbing at food items and trying to bring that food to his or her mouth. While you will still primarily be feeding your baby food which has been puréed or mashed, it is also time to start getting them in on the action. Simple finger foods which they can munch on include: pasta (macaroni and rotini cut were our preferred pasta shape and should be cooked softer than *al dente* in my opinion for easier swallowing), summer sweet peas, cooked beans, soft cheese, very soft fruit which has been cut up into small pieces, dry toast, and unsweetened oat ring cereals (eg. Multi-grain Cheerios®).

By the way, welcome to the world of Cheerios. They will be everywhere for the next few years. You can take them anywhere, they are easy for little ones to eat and have saved many moms from a child meltdown. I promise you, you will find yourself popping a few into your own mouth now and again.

Over the course of a few months, your baby will have been introduced to many new foods and flavours. You can choose to feed your baby meat and vegetable items separately at meal time or you can begin to prepare all-inclusive stews as I did. Most of my children's meals were stew-like and included some combination of all the aforementioned foods, i.e. whatever I had on hand at home.

The general recipe goes something like this:

- Boil some water in a pot.

- Add a hand-size piece of meat.

- Add 2-3 different vegetables. Typically I would use carrots because I always have carrots on hand, something green like celery, peas, zucchini or asparagus.

- Add some type of starch. I would switch it up between a ½ cup of rice or a small sized pasta (eg. Alphabet or Pastina) and/or potatoes.

- Once cooked, I would strain the food, purée or mash depending on my baby's eating development and then add some of the cooking water to bring it to the desired consistency.

Some babies refuse certain foods (eg. green vegetables) and no matter what tricks you play to get them to open their mouth, that food will inevitably come flying right back at you. By preparing foods in this manner when they were infants, I never worried that they weren't getting a balanced diet. All the good stuff was in there.

This type of meal is still a household staple except I no longer have to purée the food. You can create so many different flavours depending on the combination of meat and vegetables you choose. With a little seasoning and olive oil, it's a hearty meal for the entire family.

It can get confusing when you start your baby on solid foods. *"How much food should I prepare? What time should I feed the baby? When do I introduce different foods?"* You'll get the hang of it fairly quickly but, just in case, I have included a month-by-month sample meal plan as a reference. *"Bon appétit little one!"*

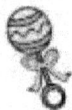

SAMPLE MEAL PLAN – 6 months	
Time of day	**What to feed**
Early morning	Breast milk or formula
Breakfast	Breast milk or formula 2–3 tbsp iron-fortified cereal mixed with breast milk, formula, or water (start with 1 tbsp at breakfast only and gradually increase portion size)
Lunch	Breast milk or formula
Mid-afternoon	Breast milk or formula
Dinner	Breast milk or formula 2–3 tbsp iron-fortified cereal mixed with breast milk, formula, or water
Night	Breast milk or formula as required

SAMPLE MEAL PLAN – 7 months	
Time of day	**What to feed**
Early morning	Breast milk or formula
Breakfast	Breast milk or formula 2–3 tbsp iron-fortified cereal mixed with breast milk, formula, or water
Lunch	Breast milk or formula 2 tbsp of fruit or vegetable
Mid-afternoon	Breast milk or formula
Dinner	Breast milk or formula 2–3 tbsp iron-fortified cereal mixed with breast milk, formula, or water
Night	Breast milk or formula as required

SAMPLE MEAL PLAN – 8 months	
Time of day	**What to feed**
Early morning	Breast milk or formula
Breakfast	Breast milk or formula 2–3 tbsp iron-fortified cereal mixed with breast milk, formula, or water
Lunch	Breast milk or formula 2 tbsp of fruit or vegetable 2 tbsp of protein-rich food (meat or alternatives)
Mid-afternoon	Breast milk or formula
Dinner	Breast milk or formula 2–3 tbsp iron-fortified cereal mixed with breast milk, formula, or water
Night	Breast milk or formula as required

SAMPLE MEAL PLAN – 9+ months	
Time of day	**What to feed**
Early morning	Breast milk or formula
Breakfast	Breast milk or formula
	2–3 tbsp iron-fortified cereal mixed with breast milk, formula, or water
Lunch	Breast milk or formula
	2 tbsp of fruit
	2 tbsp of vegetable
	2 tbsp of protein-rich food (meat or alternatives)*
Mid-afternoon	Breast milk or formula
	Snack (eg. mini-yogurt, cheese)
Dinner	Breast milk or formula
	2 tbsp of fruit
	2 tbsp of vegetable
	2 tbsp of protein-rich food (meat or alternatives)
	Finger foods (macaroni, peas, etc.)
Night	Breast milk or formula as required

*Once I had introduced my baby to all varying food choices, I started preparing the stew-like meals mentioned above which incorporated meat, vegetables and grains and would typically serve 4-6 tbsp of food (or 4-6 frozen portions).

CHAPTER 32

8 THINGS YOU UNKNOWINGLY GIVE UP WHEN YOU DECIDE TO HAVE A BABY

Here are some of the delightful things you have unknowingly given up by the mere fact that you have decided to become a mommy:

1. **Ownership of your body**

   Most of us know that when you are pregnant, for 9 months your body will be growing another human being. In order to do this, it must work harder, stretch, grow, heat up and do all sorts of things that will often leave us down-right miserable. Then that same body gives birth and in the process suffers extreme trauma. We recover from this ordeal, some quicker than others, but all the same, we think that once we give birth, we will get our bodies back. Alas, we don't.

   Over the next couple of years it will feel that someone is always pulling at you or wanting something from your body. Nursing, cuddling, bathing, co-sleeping, not to mention spouses wanting some attention too. While most of the time, it feels amazing to nurture, I will admit that there were times where I felt like screaming for everyone to stop touching me.

2. **Sleeping in**
You can just kiss this concept good-bye for several years to come. Craving sleep will become a favorite topic of discussion with other new parents. Even if you have a child that develops great sleeping habits, the post 8:00am wake-up is forever a thing of the past.

3. **Uninterrupted conversations**
Remember those days where you spent hours chatting with your significant other or your friends about anything and everything. Life with children changes that for awhile. It comes back though so don't fret. Just be patient because for a(long)while there will be interruptions due to crying, feeding, diaper changes, spit up, crying, picking up whatever has fallen (toys, food, baby), helping child discover the world, refereeing children playing together, some more crying.

4. **Spontaneous get up and go**

    Every excursion will now involve packing *stuff*. Some people practically bring their entire home with them every time they head out but even the more sensible parents quickly realize that spontaneity suffers tremendously with the arrival of a child. The day will come again when you can leave the house with your child and nothing else but in the meantime, pack the diapers, wipes, change of clothes, bottle, sippy cup, food, spoon, snacks, bib, blanket, hat, sunscreen, toys, hand sanitizer, stroller.

5. **A quiet car ride**

    Car rides will be quiet only when your baby is sleeping. The rest of the time, it will be filled with the sounds of baby toys, Fisher Price Little People CDs, Dora and Boots, and certainly some crying.

6. **A life without logistics**

    Having a baby automatically signs you up for a life full of logistics. You are constantly planning whether it's to plan a night out with your partner, or to figure out whether you can fit in some grocery shopping before baby's nap time. Having friends and family to help is fantastic especially as children continue to grow and get involved in more and more activities that require a university degree in scheduling and a personal chauffeur.

7. **Your bed**

Name one child who does not think that Mommy and Daddy's bed is the best place in the world. Any sleep issues that your child may face from nightmares to growing pains to just not being able to sleep somehow get resolved in the magic of Mommy and Daddy's bed. And no matter how big or small this bed may be your child will always somehow manage to sleep on your head.

8. **Bathroom privacy**

For years I longed for the day when I could regain my privacy in the bathroom. From the moment your baby is born, alone time in the bathroom is almost non-existent. At first, they can't get around on their own, so you may find yourself bringing them into the bathroom when you want to get ready or take a shower. Then as they start to crawl around, they barge right in there exploring, holding up tampons, whatever they can get their hands on and you're just happy they are letting you get ready. Then they go through separation anxiety and start crying the moment you walk away from them so you find yourself doing your business with a baby staring right at you or else leaving them outside the door crying the entire time; either way, not conducive to an easy time in the bathroom.

With bath time, you may find yourself taking a bath or shower with your baby and it is fascinating to see how more aware they become as the months go by. From discovering their own bodies to suddenly looking up and seeing mom or dad and getting that interesting look on their face as if they are thinking *"Hey Dad, what's that down there?"* or *"What are those Mom?"*

To this day, if my children hear the bath water running, they will come screaming outside the door, asking if they can take a bath with me. I say screaming because they are furious with me that I have started locking the bathroom door again. For years I left it open and they would always manage to appear in there the moment I walked in, or the moment I was stepping out of the shower, or bending over to apply cream on my legs, or sitting on the toilet bowl, even if they had been playing quietly before. I lost all dignity over the last few years but now it's time to reclaim some of it.

Despite all you give up when having a child there are so many more things you gain, too many to list here and too hard to describe with mere words.

CHAPTER 33

SLEEPING ON THE GO

While on maternity leave, there were so many times that I found myself alone in my car with a sleeping baby. I do mean *my* sleeping baby, not just any random sleeping baby. Having had such difficulty getting her to nap, or to stay asleep for any prolonged period of time, it would pain me to arrive at my destination and realize that she had just fallen asleep. I longed for a baby that would allow me to transfer her from car seat to stroller, or car seat to crib, without waking up but alas, it was never meant to be.

You may notice that some new moms are obsessed with feeding their little ones, always worried that they just aren't eating enough. Once we got passed the initial difficulties with breastfeeding, things were easy so it was never that big of a deal for me. On the other hand, I was absolutely nuts about sleeping and convinced that if my baby would just get some more sleep then all the crying would stop. As such, there was no way that I was going to give up this time of peace and rest for my baby *"Or for myself, who are we kidding?"*

These are some of the many scenarios that you may find yourself in while on the go with baby. What would you do?

1. You show up at a friend's house and your baby is asleep in the car. Do you wait in the car until the baby wakes up? Realize that your friends will look at you like you are odd, particularly if they have no children or if they have one of *those* children that sleeps anywhere and never cries. The dilemma of the sleep-deprived mom (and baby) is often lost on those not in the throes of it as well.

2. Your baby is asleep in the car and you are hungry. What's a mom to do? Perhaps the drive-through? The loud voice over the intercom asking "What can we get for you?" had my baby awake and in tears within seconds. *"Next time, should I just pop into a convenient store to buy a snack and leave the baby in the car?"* The paranoia about something bad happening kept me from doing this but I guarantee you that many mothers have asked themselves the same question endless times. *"For now, I guess I'll just dig*

into whatever Cheerios scraps I can find in the diaper bag."

3. You pull up at home and your baby is asleep. It's cold outside. *"Do I leave the car running? Will my baby get too cold? What am I doing to the environment? Should I just bring her inside? Maybe she won't wake up? Wrong! Shit, should have left the car running. Screw the planet!"*

4. You pull up at home and your baby is asleep. It's hot outside. *"Should I open all the windows, grab a book, pull up a chair and read close by. Will she be too hot? Will she get enough of a breeze? Should I just leave the car and A/C running?"*

These were the ramblings of a sleep-deprived mom. There were so many questions racing around in my head and it seems crazy in retrospect. It probably was. But there was something so satisfying about watching my baby sleep peacefully that I was willing to just sit there and wait it out. Too bad smart phones weren't the norm back in the *old days* (anything pre-2009). They sure would have helped pass the time.

CHAPTER 34

SAY CHEESE!

I love looking at pictures. Every so often when I visit my parents, I'll take out the old photo albums and look at the couple of hundred pictures my parents have taken over the years. I love the pictures of my parents before they had kids as well as all the goofy pictures of my brothers and I over the years. But yes, I did say there were only a couple hundred pictures. Three large photo albums to be precise. There are probably a whole bunch of doubles sitting in some storage box but they don't really count. *"Who were my parents making those double prints for anyway?"*

That is nothing in comparison to the few hundred pictures I took just last year alone. Times have sure changed and so has the technology we have at our disposal. Sometimes I question whether it is for the better as I observe the paparazzi frenzy of parents at every school concert but then again, their children will be able to relive the moment when they get older and, like I said before, I love looking at old pictures.

When you first have a baby, you quickly realize that there are so many cute things that your baby does every single day that you may find it nearly impossible not to take hundreds of pictures each day let alone over their lifetime. From the very first day, you will be fascinated with your baby's little face and those tiny little fingers and toes. In those first days, they sleep so often and I found myself just sitting and staring at that little face. I couldn't resist snapping picture after picture of my tightly swaddled sleeping baby. I could see her eyelids slightly flicker each time the flash would go on. *"Sorry little one, I'll let you sleep in peace"*.

Then there were the hundreds of pictures of her smiling, yawning, trying to lift her head when I put her on her tummy, taking a bath, eating, crawling, and playing. It is a love affair with your baby and you want to capture as much of it as you can. As your baby gets older and you move out of the honeymoon phase of being a new mom, a quick glance at any of these baby photos will bring you back to the feeling of fascination you have with your little one right now. It will shock you how quickly they change. These pictures will also serve as evidence of how in love you are with your child when they one day proclaim *"You are the worst mommy in the world and you never loved me"*. *"Wait a second! Of course I love you. Look at these pictures. Do you see? There's your proof!"*

Everything is possible when you look at that sweet innocence. If you are ever feeling a little sad, just look at any of these pictures. It's free therapy, I promise. To those not going through the same baby experience as you, all the picture-taking (or picture-*sharing*) seems excessive but don't let that bother you. My one piece of advice however is to get yourself in some of those pictures as well. Moms are always the first to grab the camera and capture everyone else in those special moments but so rarely do we place ourselves in the spotlight. When they are older, your children will want to see you in those shots with them. They won't care or even notice whether your hair was washed, whether you were in a ratty T-shirt, or whether you had lost all the baby weight. So stop over-analyzing what you look like, grab that little bundle of love and pass the camera to someone else for once. *"Say cheese!"*

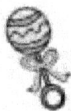

CHAPTER 35

HOW I PICTURED MATERNITY LEAVE

Women from around the world face many different challenges when they have babies and I am fortunate to live in Canada, a country where parents are given the opportunity to take up to a one year leave of absence from their work to care for a newborn. Women are eligible for a 17-week paid maternity leave and then either the mother or father can take an additional 35 weeks of parental leave and still be guaranteed their job (or an equivalent job) upon their return to work. Could it be better? Probably. Could it be worse? Hell yes. I'm not however looking to debate what benefits women should be eligible for but, more importantly, to fill you in on the possibility that a pending long-term leave of absence from work may lead to severe delusional thought. Let me explain.

I was pregnant with my first child and if I could just hang on for a few more months at work with all this nausea business, I was going to have an entire year without work. Let's just stop and think about this for a minute. I was going to have the entire summer off. When was the last time that happened? High school? And it wasn't just the summer that I would have off, all four seasons would come and go and only then would I go back to work. It's crazy, right? *"Woo hoo! Vacation time! This is going to be amazing!"*

By this point of the book, even if you are not already going through it, you should still have a pretty clear picture of what life will be like during your baby's first year. None of that real stuff factored into my vision. Suffice it to say, that vision of maternity leave couldn't have been further from the truth.

To all my American friends, I am so sorry but honestly, how do you get your shit together to head back to work after six weeks? At the six-week mark post-partum, I was firmly locked in a vortex of breastfeeding, colic, abdominal pain, sleep deprivation, and dark circles. Not exactly what I had been fantasizing about when I was pregnant. Feel free to laugh or think me a fool. It's embarrassing to admit but the prospect of having an entire year with no work was like a drug, leading to uncontrollable hallucinations. Here are some of my pre-baby delusions.

- My baby would spend most of her day quietly sleeping. Quiet and sleeping are definitely not two adjectives that described my baby.

- There would be plenty of time to exercise regularly and get back into shape. Instead, each time I tried walking on the treadmill I got shin splints and my pelvis would get sore. I could count the number of times I exercised during that year on my hands (maybe even just one hand).

- I would meet up regularly with friends and colleagues over lunch or coffee and bring along my perfect baby. This did work out on occasion but for the most part, my life was now defined by my baby's schedule which surprisingly enough didn't mesh well with the schedule of my working friends.

- My inner Martha Stewart would emerge and I would organize my home, sort through the basement, throw out any junk, and colour coordinated boxes would store everything else. I did eventually do this however it took me three years and a second maternity leave to finally complete.

- And the most ridiculous idea of all was that I would have enough time to register for and complete an MBA. I don't even know how to explain this one. I must have been smoking crack.

It seems that my entire vision centred around all the things I could do while this baby was sleeping. These are the silly things you may believe if you're one of the first in your circle of friends to have children. I hope I have made it clear though. There may be some time to focus on yourself during your maternity leave but it will usually amount to just enough time to shower and brush your teeth or to take a quick nap. You can't have both. And that's just perfect.

CHAPTER 36

MORE STUFF I FORGOT TO MENTION

A few more random things have just popped into my head and I feel I should give you the heads up.

1. Sometimes you will be out with your baby and they will poo and you will have either forgotten or run out of diapers. You will feel terrible. Don't. Every parent has left their baby in a dirty diaper for longer than they should have at some point.

2. Newborns get boogers, and they are not always the runny kind. You will have to suck those bad boys out of their nostrils. No, not with your mouth! With a little nasal aspirator contraption. Pick one with a tip that is fairly long and pointy so that you can fit it into the tiny nostril. When you unplug your babies blocked nose it will be disgusting and gratifying at the same time.

3. After about six months, you will realize that the interaction between you and your baby is becoming less and less one-sided and then one day you realize that you have this little buddy around who is always smiling and excited to see you.

4. The gummy smile of a baby is the best smile in the world. The two bottom teeth smile is a pretty close second.

5. Speaking of teeth, keep your glasses away from your baby. Their teeth are so sharp that it only takes a few seconds before those lenses are full of scratches. Technicians should have brought some babies into the laboratory when they were testing scratch resistant coating for lenses.

6. You can get pregnant while nursing. If you don't want to get pregnant right away, don't count on this as your form of contraception since there is no way to predict when you will begin to ovulate after giving birth.

7. If you have older children, you will be shocked at how enormous they are when you see them for the first time after giving birth.

8. Don't be surprised if you catch your older child trying to *breastfeed* a doll. The intense focus with

which my daughter was trying to hold up her shirt and keep her doll in place at the same time was both adorable and bizarre.

9. How did new parents find answers before the internet?

CHAPTER 37

BACK TO WORK ALREADY?

If you choose to work once you have children, and let's face it, most women do, depending on where you live in the world, heading back to work can happen anytime from a few weeks to several years after giving birth. In my case, my baby was a year old when I slipped on those pantyhose once again, put on my suit, and headed out the door with tears in my eyes.

Many people thought I would be itching to get back to work and while I admit that I love the feeling of accomplishment and the sense of power work provides me, leaving my little one, who was on the cusp of walking, in the care of someone else was heartbreaking. Despite how hard baby's first year can be, my daughter and I were in the throes of a love affair and I didn't want to share her. But share her I did.

As the end of my maternity leave grew closer and closer, just the thought of leaving made me nauseous. Luckily I eased into it with the help of my mother and mother-in-law. For the first few months they would alternate staying at our place to take care of their granddaughter which allowed me the flexibility to get myself back up to speed at work and not worry about drop-offs and pick-ups. This was the best option for us. It was also our only option because we couldn't find a daycare center that had an opening and we weren't interested in having a live-in nanny.

If you do plan on going back to work after giving birth and do not have family who can help with childcare, my advice to you is to start looking for care as soon as possible. Ask friends. Get recommendations. Put your name on waiting lists. In a nutshell, it can be hard to find openings and quite expensive. Our oldest daughter was placed on a centralized waiting list in early 2005 and all these years later, we have never received a call about potential openings.

Every family has their own criteria when looking for appropriate childcare but here are some things to keep in mind:

• The safety of your child should be pretty high up on that list of priorities. Finding a person or a center that genuinely cares for the well-being of these little ones that have been entrusted to them is vital. Tune in to your *Spidey* senses. You will be able to tell that some see this as a business, some are looking to make some extra cash while raising their own children but aren't that into the whole idea of a daycare, and some genuinely care about your child's well-being and development.

- Your personality may not click with that of the potential caregiver. If you don't feel comfortable with them from the get go, it probably won't get any better. We once spoke with a caregiver who was just getting her home business underway. This was for before- and after-school care and we immediately felt that it was a great fit. Unfortunately there were no more spots available. The following day we got a telephone call informing us that the spot was now available. It turns out that caregivers also want to ensure a proper fit and she was concerned about the demands of one of the families she had interviewed with. *"Sucks to be them. Yay for us!"*

- Some parents are rude to caregivers. Having witnessed this many times, I could never understand what these parents were looking to achieve. Be vocal about any concerns but being rude is just plain dumb. *"Aren't you aware that caregivers can tell when you don't respect them? Why would you look down on people responsible for caring for your child? You do realize that when you walk out the door and leave your kid there, the caregiver will still remember that you just spoke to them like they were an idiot?"*

- Having family care for your child is a great option because there is already an emotional attachment to your child but it could also cause conflict or tension if you and the family member have differing parenting styles. It may also limit the amount of interaction your child has with other children. *"And make for one demanding child if grandma or grandpa managed to lose their backbone over the years."*

- Finding care for infants is particularly difficult. Although it varies depending on where you live, the government approved ratio of children to caregiver at that young age is typically so low forcing centers to hire and maintain more staff. This can be challenging or not cost effective so many daycare centers choose to only offer care for children who are at least 12 months old and some even 18 months+.

- If there is no government subsidized childcare available where you live, any type of paid childcare service will be expensive. Monthly rates drop as your child gets older but not by any substantial amount.

- When budgeting for care, a home daycare is typically the least expensive option. Assuming an average monthly rate of $800, a family can expect to pay over $38,000 for full-time care for one child over a period of 4 years. Depending on what age your child starts school, this amount can be even higher. Licensed centers and nanny care will run you even more. Even with the help we had from grandparents, we have paid close to $80,000 for childcare for our two daughters. And it's not over yet.

- It is almost guaranteed that your child will get sick shortly after you put them in any type of care involving other children. So will you. This cycle will repeat itself many times throughout the year until you both develop some immunity.

  It seemed like my youngest had snot dripping from her nose for about six months once she started daycare. Most centers will accept a child with a cold but all bets are off if vomiting and diarrhea are involved. They typically won't allow your child back in the center for at least 48 hours after the last explosive episode which poses the challenge of finding alternate care if you are unable to take the time off work yourself. This is when parents start lying.

Despite the fact that we eased into childcare for both our daughters with the help of family, it did not reduce the amount of tears I was subjected to when I left in the morning. *"Mommy loves you baby girl but I have to go to work now. We have been glued at the hip for the last year but now it's time for you to explore the world a little bit by yourself. You are a brave little girl and I know you will do great. Don't forget that I will always be there to make sure you are safe. Now stop crying!"*

The joy on their faces however, when I walked back in at the end of the workday, took my breath away. There is nothing quite like the feeling you experience witnessing the sheer happiness in your child's face at the sight of you. But be forewarned, the moment you walk back into your house after working all day, the marathon begins. From preparing dinner to feeding your child, feeding yourself, hopefully playing a bit, bathing your child, and getting them ready for bed. It's all a whirlwind of activity. And once they are asleep is when everything else gets done, the laundry, the dishes, the emails, all that *stuff*.

Those first years require a lot of heavy lifting. There is a lot to do now. Someone else depends on us so we willingly do it all because it is not just about us anymore.

We are mothers. And we wouldn't have it any other way.

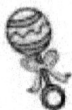

INDEX

INDEX